Contents

Acknowledgements

No book is written without help and support from others. I would particularly like to thank Dr Noel Collins, MB BS (Hons), MRCPsych who read, corrected and commented upon the chapter 'About Dementia' and Dr Doug Brown, Director of Research and Development, Alzheimer's Society who gave specific comments on the paragraphs about genetics in that chapter. Dr Gillian Nienaber, BA Hons, BSc Hons, CinPsychD, gave me help with the research and information generally. Karen Woodger RN(MH), MSc Counselling & Psychotherapy and Janice Cresdee IOSH, Registered Team Manager at Surrey County Council, both gave me valuable information about Care plans, as did Amanda Emerson also of Surrey County Council.

As with my previous books, my thanks are due to Janet Baylis and Andrew Holland at Alzheimer's Society Dementia Knowledge Centre who once again gave me an enormous amount of help to find relevant research papers and books and other useful information. The Dementia Knowledge Centre is open to anyone via Alzheimer's Society website and is a great resource for anyone interested in learning more about dementia: www.alzheimers.org.uk/dementiacatalogue

I would also like to give special thanks to my editor Georgina Bentliff who has been a source of great technical support, much encouragement and endless patience, always.

My friends and family have been very helpful in supplying and giving me permission to use the case history examples and I certainly could not have completed the book without their encouragement, the support of my two sons, Tristram and Rauf, and the many practical suggestions of my daughter-in-law, Erica Arnold.

Introduction

You may be wondering what led me to write this book. I work to support people with dementia and their families. When people are first referred to me they generally have one of two reactions. Either they thank me and say they will contact me 'when they need me' and go away – or they come to me in complete bewilderment and anxiety, unsure what I can do to help but believing that, as the doctor has referred them, they are doing the right thing.

In fact, as I point out in this book, doctors can only help so much following a diagnosis of dementia. The truth is that medication is of limited use. This does not mean that it is not worth trying – indeed, I am in favour of anyone who may possibly benefit at least trying to see if one of the 'memory drugs' can help. When faced with a devastating disease for which we have no known cure, why would you not try whatever modern medicine has to offer – particularly as the side effects to this medication are usually minor and can be stopped at once by discontinuing the drug?

I believe that at this present time the most important thing that can be offered to people who have been confronted by the 'D word' – whether as a carer or as someone who has just been diagnosed – is support. When people ask me what my job is, this is how I like to sum it up: 'I offer support.' I have been most fortunate in that my job role is defined in such a way that I am often able to 'tailor' that support to what individuals require.

However, I can only spread my support so far. In many areas of the UK, dementia support workers like myself are able to give this support, but still, it is not enough. Through this book I hope to spread the support and advice, the knowledge and expertise that I and my colleagues have accumulated, a little wider and further. Even if you do not have access to a dementia support worker through the Alzheimer's Society, you can get ideas, advice, information and support through this book.

You can read this book straight through or you can dip in and out as you feel the need. You will find a certain amount of repetition because some advice and information is relevant to many areas of care and concern. Where areas overlap I have referenced and directed readers back or forward to other chapters. There is also a handy reference section to which you can turn for further, or more in-depth, information on individual subjects.

What is dementia?

Chapter 1 begins by describing what dementia really is, for those who wish to know. 'Dementia' is not the same as Alzheimer's disease, although many people use the terms interchangeably – 'dementia' is a symptom of many conditions, of which Alzheimer's disease is the commonest, closely followed by 'vascular dementia'. This book deals with dementia from all the common causes because, as the symptoms progress, there are very few differences between them, though many differences between individuals, whatever the cause.

Chapter 1 also talks about some of the risk factors for dementia. We do not yet know what causes one person to develop the condition whilst others are spared, but we do understand some of the factors which raise the risk of any single person developing dementia. This chapter also helps someone who may be worried about their cognitive ability to differentiate between the normal mild cognitive impairment which is common in older people and true dementia. Only a doctor can diagnose the condition, but this chapter may help you to decide whether you should talk to your doctor about your memory or any related problems.

Not everyone wants to go into great detail about what dementia is or the path it is likely to follow, so some people may be tempted to skip chapter 1. For this reason I have highlighted in bold some facts that are important and which it is useful for you to really understand. If you do not wish to read in depth about what dementia is and how it may progress, you can just read the paragraphs written in bold type and have enough knowledge to help you understand the path ahead of you.

Why it helps to accept help

My advice starts in chapter 2 by suggesting that you build a team to help you. If you are caring for someone in the early stages of dementia, you may find it hard to understand why this advice comes so early in the book. However, as I explain later (see page 21), when it comes to dementia you cannot 'go it alone'. Dementia is progressive and as it progresses the carer needs help in order to help the one with dementia. It is precisely the people who believe that they will not need help and support who should read this chapter with care.

At this point I would like to refer back to what I have said at the beginning of this introduction. There are people who refuse support at the time of diagnosis. Of course they are entitled to do that and no one would wish to force unwanted advice on them, or to interfere in the lives of any other person. I know, however, that I can give the best help in the early stages and am always pleased when I can work with people straight after diagnosis. Then I can give them the greatest opportunities to help themselves and to make small adjustments so that, as dementia progresses, they are in a better position to cope in their own way. In particular, people with dementia who live alone and accept support when needed are more likely to be able to continue living in their own home for longer and have a good quality of life while doing so.

So perhaps, if you are one of those who prefers not to accept the services of a dementia adviser, or a community psychiatric nurse, or a social care worker, you will find this book particularly useful because it encapsulates, I hope, all the advice and support I give to those with whom I work.

There are many people who could be part of your team of supporters and each team will be different as each person with dementia is different. Perhaps the most important point about building your team is the simple suggestion that you *ask* others to help you, and that you also ask them to do specific things so they understand how they can help. Most of us really like to feel of use to others and to help those who need this, so no one should hold back from asking for help and support from their friends, neighbours and colleagues. Health and social care professionals are part of the caring team too and it is important to ask them for help when you need it.

How the professionals can help you

You will find that many new people enter your lives along with the diagnosis of dementia – many of these are health and social care professionals and in chapter 3 I try to explain the role of these individuals and how they can help you in your dementia journey. There are many new terms to learn as well – 'care plan', 'carer's assessment', 're-ablement', 'occupational therapy'. It can be unnerving to deal with professionals who, although kind and well meaning, do not explain their role in your life.

I begin chapter 3 by discussing the sometimes difficult task of actually getting a diagnosis. People who are worried about their memory may well avoid going to the doctor and, as I explain, many people in the early stages of dementia are actually NOT worried about their memory. They may think instead that the people around them are being difficult or bad tempered and less understanding than in the past. Nor is it a simple thing to ask a GP to 'test' someone's memory or check up on their cognition. Doctors are only too aware of the confidentiality which exists in the patient/doctor relationship and they will seldom discuss the situation, even with a spouse or life partner. In chapter 3 I also explain the steps that may be made and the tests which can lead to a diagnosis.

You are likely to become more familiar with the inside of doctors' consulting rooms and the hospitals than you would like. It is therefore useful to know the role of the different health professionals and how they will be able to help you. Awareness of dementia is improving, but you will still meet with much ignorance and it can help to know how to handle matters and explain things so that you can be of most help to the person you care for.

Understanding how behaviour changes

When people think about dementia, they usually think of confused behaviour and aggression. Indeed, many of the people I help to support worry that aggressive behaviour will arise even if the person they care for has always been calm and peaceable. There are many challenges that arise when people are confused and unable to do the things they have always been able to do, but very often managing this is all about knowing the right approach and understanding what is causing the person with dementia to be upset. As I explain later on (see page 97), it is important to understand how thinking changes in someone with dementia. Logical and structured thought is affected quite early in the condition's development, while emotional thought is retained. The person with dementia may not understand what you are trying to tell them, but they will certainly understand your feelings about it. If you remain calm and understanding they will be reassured, whereas if you get anxious and upset they will begin to become anxious themselves, and because they are unable to rationalise that anxiety they may behave in ways that seem strange and illogical.

Some kinds of unusual behaviour are more common than others and I have tried to explain the times and occasions when these behaviours are more likely and to give suggestions about how you might manage these. Because dementia is progressive you may not feel at the time of diagnosis that this chapter applies in your case, but it will be reassuring to have the information to hand when you might need it. It can also help just to know that you are not alone in experiencing what doctors often call 'challenging behaviour' from the person you care for. Talking to others in your situation can help to make you feel more comfortable about looking after someone with dementia.

Understanding how communication changes

Communication problems are one of the first symptoms of many dementias and it can take carers some time to realise that the problem for the person with dementia lies not just in making themselves understood but also in understanding what others say to them. These difficulties can make social situations very stressful, and by the time dementia is diagnosed it may be that the person concerned has already withdrawn from many activities and relationships because they find social intercourse too hard to sustain. However, a good and varied social life and interaction with others are most important in slowing the progression of dementia. There is ample research showing that people who keep up their friendships and their social contacts live a more fulfilling life despite their memory problems.

Chapter 5 looks at communication problems in depth, examines ways to ease the difficulties and gives you some specific hints – and even narratives – to help you adjust your conversation and speech so that you give the best support you can to the person you care for. Most people with dementia really want to communicate with others, to tell how they feel and to continue to bear their part in conversations, and if you can assist them in this you will be doing a great service.

Understanding why your behaviour needs to change

Many carers ask me how they can get the person they care for to change their behaviour to make life easier or to make things more acceptable to others. All of them are surprised when I explain that they cannot change the behaviour of the person with dementia. You see, the changes to the brain which happen in dementia mean that it is very difficult indeed, if not impossible, for someone with dementia to learn anything new – and that includes behavioural adaptations. On the contrary, it is carers who need to change the way they behave if they are to continue to lead a happy and companionable life with the one they care for.

Most of us find it hard to accept this truth. The person with dementia is often seen to be acting irrationally and making life difficult for those around them. Carers think that if they could just get the person with dementia to understand how they affect others and to change the way they behave it would make life run more smoothly – and no doubt it would. Sadly, it can't happen.

Relationships without dementia involve give and take, even if they are never entirely equal. With dementia, the ability to 'give' goes and the person with dementia cannot do anything about this – the carer does all the giving and the person with dementia seems to do all the taking. There are, however, ways of making this unavoidable situation less stressful for both carer and cared-for. The carer has to remember that in order to make adaptations in behaviour it is necessary to be able to reason, to think things out and to plan ahead. People with dementia gradually lose these abilities. If you can truly come to terms with this – and it is not easy – life becomes calmer and less stressed. There are ways to cope and ways to adapt and I show you some of those ways.

How to preserve independence

One of the best ways we can help someone with dementia is to assist them to live their lives to the full and this involves allowing them to be as independent as possible. It gets harder to do this as the dementia progresses and the ingenuity of care-givers is often challenged. No one wants to be entirely dependent upon others and the realisation that this dependency is growing each day can make people who have dementia very frustrated and angry. This dependency encompasses not just tasks which need to be thought through or planned, but gradually includes even the simplest of activities, such as reading a magazine or watching a TV programme. Everyday life becomes more difficult and more frustrating for someone struggling to live with dementia.

There are many tried and tested ways to help and support someone in this quest for as much independence as possible. Sadly, people who have dementia often find the best efforts of their nearest and dearest annoying and irritating and carers can be demoralised and deeply upset when their offers of help are rejected and their attempts at support scorned. This is the time to enlist the help of your 'team' and to allow others to take a hand. There are many ways that your team can help and there are many simple steps that can make a huge difference – such as breaking a task down into its component parts, reminding people of the next step at critical moments and, above all, giving enough time so that a brain which is no longer functioning as it once did can have the chance to find its way, in its own time, giving the person with dementia a sense of satisfaction and achievement.

Even small, everyday tasks become harder for those with dementia and helping them to cope with the small skills of everyday living can be challenging. Chapter 8 gives carers many tips on how to 'step up' their support as the dementia progresses and shows how to incorporate help from others, including incorporating respite time in day centres into your plan for caring. Many people resist the idea of a day centre, thinking of it as a 'dumping ground', or as demeaning for the person with dementia. Once you read the comments from those who have dementia and who enjoy the day centre (see page 14), and once you are able to understand that the day centre provides an uncritical and stress-free environment (provided of course that you choose the right day centre), you will change your mind and realise the value of this time for both the carer and the person with dementia.

How to delay dementia

Coping with dementia on a daily basis is one thing, but often people ask me if there is anything they, or the person they care for, can do to modify or even slow down the progress of the dementia. There is solid research which shows that certain lifestyle changes – such as increasing exercise, improving nutrition and keeping up social contacts and interaction with others – is of benefit in allowing someone with dementia to live as independently and to have as much enjoyment of life as possible.

I believe that in the future much more attention will be paid to this kind of 'self help' activity and that care professionals, doctors and nurses, as well as dementia support workers, will be actively involved in pointing people towards rewarding social activities and showing them how to keep up lifestyle behaviours which slow the progress of dementia and allow people to live an active and rewarding life whatever their cognitive ability. Professional care-givers will move away from only providing the 'passive' care-giving activities of keeping people clean and fed and comfortable, and move towards helping them to increase their enjoyment of life and of the 'here and now' in which they live. Because the 'executive function' of the brain (that is, planning, decision-making and logical thought) is one of the first areas of ability to be lost in most types of dementia, the part played by carers will be vital in this area of care and support.

For those carers reading this book as a source of information and support, I have included brief notes on nutritional factors that research points to as being significant. Much of this research is still ongoing, but provided you keep to accepted guidelines you are unlikely to do harm by making changes in the diet and including certain dietary supplements. Also included are many suggestions of ways to increase the amount of exercise in the life of the person for whom you are caring and to do this in a way that will be enjoyable and pleasant. Readers of my book, *The Essential Guide to Avoiding Dementia*, will be able to pinpoint the research behind these tips.

Practical matters

Two chapters (10 and 11) in this book deal with essentially practical matters. It seems that health professionals and others often forget that those with dementia can suffer from the same minor, and sometimes major, health problems that can affect any older person. Understanding when someone with dementia is ill or in pain may be more difficult as their ability to communicate is gradually reduced. I have therefore tried to give readers advice and information on recognising illness and understanding how to help the person they care for when visiting the doctor or during hospital stays. Equally, I give guidance on recognising the roles of different health professionals and knowing when their help is useful and important.

There are other practical things which many of us avoid thinking about or acting upon. However, we would all be wise to plan for the future, and the time after a diagnosis is a time for taking stock and for carrying out some of the practical actions which will make life easier in the future and give our loved ones comfort and reassurance. Everyone should make a Will, and it is a very sensible action to arrange to give lasting power of attorney to someone we trust so that, if the time comes when we can no longer manage our financial or welfare affairs, then at least we can have confidence that they will be handled in the way we would wish. People often think that authorising a power of attorney means relinquishing all authority, but giving power of attorney is a 'rainy day' action – something like taking out insurance – a 'just in case' action which means that we have given thought to the problems which might face those we love in the future.

There are other financial practicalities which may have to be dealt with. The State gives only limited financial help to those with dementia since it is presently considered to be a social problem rather than a medical one, but some benefits and allowances are claimable and – as in many other situations – those who are completely unable to pay after assessment by the social care team will be given the financial assistance they need. The benefits system is a complex 'minefield' but there are organisations (such as Citizens' Advice Bureaux) that will help you to find your way through this. Some people also like to plan in case the need should arise for residential care in a 'care home' and this is a sensible idea.

If the worst happens and someone with dementia has to be admitted to hospital, it can be helpful to have considered this possibility beforehand and to have a written statement of likes, dislikes and personal preferences to which hospital staff can refer in order to make the stay in hospital more bearable. Several versions of this kind of statement, sometime called a 'hospital passport', can be obtained from your support worker, from health professionals or by downloading the document from websites such as www.alzheimers.org.uk. Carers and people with dementia can complete this document together and keep it safely against the time it may be needed.

Some people would wish to think more deeply about possible future scenarios and there is information in this section of the book (see page 191) on practical matters relating to Advance Decisions and end-of-life wishes.

How to look after yourself

I have included a final – and most important – chapter that discusses the needs of the carer. Caring for someone else can be very rewarding and many of us are glad to 'give something back', but caring can also be very stressful and it can seem very lonely. It is easy to become isolated and to feel that no one else can understand the burden that we bear. In this final chapter, I urge care-givers to understand the importance of thinking about their own needs and comforts, because looking after their own health and well-being is vital. It is not selfish to consider your own health. Apart from anything else, the well-being of the person you care for depends upon your ability to carry out that care. There is a variety of help available in the community and you should not feel guilty about accessing that help and accepting any support offered. Nor should you feel guilty about asking for help. If this book can reassure you about that and point you to sources of support, it has achieved its aim.

If you are not in England

All my experience of helping those with dementia, be it professional or personal, has been in relation to England. Practical details – for example, in relation to Lasting Power of Attorney – therefore are specific to England. However, the PRINCIPLES – for example, provisionally handing over responsibility for your financial affairs in the event of loss of competence BEFORE you lose that competence – are the same for any person facing the diagnosis of dementia. Please do therefore read the chapters on practical matters, not for the detail so much as for the generic guidance which should stand translation to any part of the Western world. You will also find that I have included sources of information for other regions/countries, notably Scotland and the Republic of Ireland.

Learning from my readers

I have learned most of what is in this book from those I help with dementia. As a reader facing those same problems, please do let me know if you think there are ways this book could be improved and topics that should be added. Send your feedback to info@adaptdementia.com.

Mary Jordan

Chapter 1

About dementia

If someone close to you has been given a diagnosis of dementia you are likely to be going through a range of emotions. Some people find themselves wanting to find out all they can – others would rather not know more than the bare facts. This chapter tells you about dementia and has been written in such a way that, if you like, you can just read the short headings and get the minimum of information. If, on the other hand, you would like to understand much more, you can read the whole chapter thoroughly and then do your own further research.

Even if you prefer not to know everything at this stage, I recommend that you read the short paragraphs in bold: this will help your understanding and mean that you can care for the person with the diagnosis as well as possible.

What do we mean by 'dementia'?

The word dementia is an umbrella term that covers a number of neurological degenerative conditions including Alzheimer's disease, vascular dementia and fronto-temporal dementia.

Given the 'D' word is one that frightens people a lot, it is important we understand what it means. Sometimes the popular press seems to have a problem separating 'dementia' from Alzheimer's disease. Dementia is a word that describes the symptoms that develop in a number of different diseases. There are thought to be more than 200 types of dementia and Alzheimer's disease is only one of them, although it is believed to be the most common, affecting rather more than half of those with symptoms of dementia. The next most common form of dementia is thought to be vascular dementia.

Dementia with Lewy bodies (or Lewy body dementia) and fronto-temporal dementia are two other types. The term 'fronto-temporal dementia' is in itself used to describe a range of conditions, including Pick's disease, frontal lobe degeneration and the dementia associated with motor neurone disease, where damage occurs in the frontal or temporal lobe areas of the brain, or both.

There are many other rarer causes of dementia. Dementia may also occur as a result of other specific diseases (for example, in Huntington's disease). These will not be covered in any detail in this book.

You may also hear the term **mild cognitive impairment (MCI)**. This is not dementia but rather a condition where someone may have some of the features of dementia (mainly memory problems – see below) but the person affected is able to function in their daily life (see also pages 9–10). It is thought that people with MCI have a higher risk of developing dementia later on.

Dementia, therefore, can be described as a collection of symptoms, including memory loss, perceived personality change, and impaired intellectual functions resulting from degenerative disease or trauma to the brain. These changes are not part of normal ageing and they are severe enough to impact daily living, independence and relationships. This book is about coping with dementia, whatever its cause, as the long-term challenges are the same, as I describe later in this chapter. It is, however, principally about dementia caused by Alzheimer's disease, vascular dementia, dementia with Lewy bodies and fronto-lobal dementia. Much that I have included is relevant to rarer causes but I do not look at these specifically.

Chapter 1

What is the difference between dementia and normal ageing?

With dementia, someone is likely to show a noticeable decline in the ability to communicate, to learn skills, to remember things and to solve problems – what is known as 'executive function'.

These changes may occur quickly or very slowly over time. If you think someone may have dementia you may have noticed some or all of the following:

- Short-term memory loss
- Impaired judgement
- Difficulties with abstract thinking
- Faulty reasoning
- Inappropriate behaviour
- Loss of communication skills
- Disorientation in time and place
- Gait, motor and balance problems
- Neglect of personal care and safety
- Hallucinations, abnormal beliefs, anxiety, agitation.

My mother-in-law suddenly became very frightened of being alone in the house. She double-locked all the doors, which at first we thought a sensible precaution. But later we found she had put chairs under the door handles as well, to prevent them being opened and she started getting very worried when we left the house and began ringing us up at all hours to check where we were.

The fact is that, as we grow older, many of us suffer from some of the above symptoms. It is very difficult for someone without medical knowledge to know whether these are a sign of 'normal' ageing or are evidence of developing dementia. It can be very frightening to forget your telephone number or a recent event and then to worry that you are developing dementia.

> *Looking back I remember when our first grandchild was born – a boy. We were both delighted but for some reason my husband kept referring to the baby as 'she' – even though he was called Michael. I dismissed it as a slip of the tongue at the time, although he kept on doing it. Now I wonder if that was the first 'sign'.*

Dementia is not part of normal ageing. Older people may have memory lapses but the memory problems associated with dementia are specific to the illness.

Losing your thread

It is possible to compare some of the symptoms and to see how these differ in normal ageing and in dementia. For example, any elderly (or not so elderly) person may complain about memory loss, but on questioning they would be able to provide examples of this, such as 'I completely forgot where I put my keys yesterday.' However, someone with dementia may not even realise that they have memory problems, may indeed vigorously deny this and may accuse others of making things up when they are given examples of how they have forgotten something.

Most people have occasions when they have to search for a word or substitute a word temporarily. Someone with dementia frequently has to pause to find the right word and may often lose their way in a sentence, perhaps trailing off or diverting to some other subject or drifting into irrelevance.

I noticed my sister would lose track of herself in the middle of a sentence. We had always had very lively discussions about many subjects but she started losing the thread of an argument. If I prompted her she would make an excuse and say I was distracting her or that she couldn't be bothered to talk because she was tired.

Getting lost in familiar places

As we get older some of us may find we have to pause to recall directions clearly or may have to repeat directions to remember them, but we do not get lost in familiar places or forget the route home from the local shops, for example. People with dementia may often get lost in familiar places. Many carers say one of the first things they noticed was that the person with dementia forgot a simple route, such as the way back from the toilet in a restaurant (this is a very good example of short-term memory loss).

Forgetting what just happened

Older people generally can remember recent personal events, especially major events, but people with dementia may forget what happened yesterday even if it was something as important as a grandchild's christening. They may, however, easily recall events in the distant past with great clarity.

My father kept accusing us of neglecting him and not coming to see him. If I pointed out that we had come to see him the day before, he would strongly deny this and even get abusive. Sometimes I could convince him by showing something I had brought with me on a previous visit but often he would accuse me of tricking him or 'planting the evidence' just to catch him out.

Losing interest

People with dementia may lose interest in social activities or hobbies and pastimes. They may forget to wash or be unable to put on a simple article of clothing.

Older people generally retain their social skills and normal routines, such as washing and dressing, even if it takes them longer to carry out these actions than when they were younger. They also usually continue to enjoy social occasions and their normal interests.

The first thing I recall noticing was that he stopped going fishing. Previously it had been his favourite hobby. He often talked about going but he didn't actually do anything. If I asked him about it he usually had an excuse – he was busy, or something had come up that was more important. It was only much later that I looked back and saw that as the first sign.

What else might it be?

These signs and symptoms are indicative of dementia, but we have to be wary of making assumptions. For example, some forms of **depression** cause people to lose interest in their appearance and to cease bothering to wash or change their clothes. There are also a number of conditions that may 'mimic' dementia or cause a temporary dementia-like state. One example is **low blood sugar**, which can cause susceptible people to become confused and agitated. A **urinary infection** can also cause symptoms similar to dementia in older people. These symptoms normally come on fairly suddenly, without the history of a slow decline that we usually see with developing dementia.

WHY ME?

We do not know the cause(s) of dementia but we understand what some of the risk factors are. Having a number of risk factors may make you more likely to develop dementia.

We do not know an absolute 'cause' of dementia. Research seems to indicate that, as with many diseases, there is no one cause, but there are a number of 'risk factors' which might increase the risk of dementia developing in any one person.

It is believed that the risk of developing dementia is affected by a combination of genetic and environmental factors. This suggests that everyone is at risk of developing dementia but some are more at risk than others. Because a specific cause is not known it is also true to say that we do not know what factors do not cause dementia. However, research indicates that it is not a contagious disease – that is, you cannot 'catch' dementia from being with someone who develops the disease.

Age as a risk factor

It is important to remember that dementia is NOT a normal symptom of ageing. However, age is the most significant known risk factor for dementia. It is possible to develop dementia early in life (early-onset dementia), but the chances of developing it increase significantly as we get older. One in 50 people between the ages of 65 and 70 has some form of dementia, compared with one in five people over the age of 80.

Other risk factors include uncontrolled or poorly controlled diabetes, past injuries to the head, genetic makeup, and some other specific medical conditions.

Genetic risk factors for early-onset dementia

Certain genes can affect a person's risk of developing Alzheimer's disease specifically, although our knowledge about this is incomplete. **The evidence of a genetic cause is stronger for early-onset dementia.**

The three genes that have a major effect on the risk of developing early-onset Alzheimer's disease are, for those who want the detail, the amyloid precursor protein (APP) gene and two presenilin genes (PSEN-1 and PSEN-2). People with abnormalities in these genes can develop the disease in their 30s or 40s, and usually come from families in which several members also have early-onset Alzheimer's disease.

Genetic mutations on these three genes are very rare: they account for fewer than one in 1,000 cases of Alzheimer's disease.

It is believed that everyone who inherits a genetic defect in any one of the three genes will develop Alzheimer's disease at a comparatively early age. And, on average, half of the children of a person with one of these rare genetic defects will inherit the disease. Those who do not inherit the defective genes cannot pass it on.

If you have two or more close relatives (a close relative is defined as a parent or sibling) who developed Alzheimer's disease before the age of 60, you could ask your doctor to advise you about genetic counselling and testing.

Genetic risks for late-onset dementia

With late-onset dementia, the genetics are not so clear. For example, a gene called apolipoprotein E (ApoE) has been shown to play a part in the development of late-onset Alzheimer's disease and possibly also in vascular dementia. The effects of various combinations of the ApoE gene seem to be subtle and, although it is not believed that the gene directly causes Alzheimer's, the variations seem to increase or decrease the risk of developing the disease.

As research on the genetics of Alzheimer's disease progresses, researchers are uncovering links between late-onset Alzheimer's and a number of other genes, including CLU, PICALM, CR1, BIN1, ABCA7, MS4A, CD33, EPHA1 and CD2AP. These genes appear to have a much smaller effect than ApoE on the risk of developing Alzheimer's disease, but research has shown that they may be significant. Research to find further genes which increase the risk or have a protective effect is very much ongoing and it is possible that new information about genes linked to dementia will in time give us a better understanding of the biological mechanisms and potential future treatments for dementia.

'Mild cognitive impairment' as a risk factor

Mild cognitive impairment (MCI) is not dementia, but anyone with MCI is more likely to develop dementia.

MCI is a relatively new expression in medical terminology. It is a descriptive term rather than a specific medical condition or disease and describes the memory loss that the sufferer – and those around them – will have become aware of. Formal memory tests may highlight this memory loss but the person will not have any other symptoms of dementia.

People with MCI usually have impaired memory or mild impairments in other areas of brain function, such as planning or attention span, but do not experience significant problems in carrying out the functions of everyday living.

It is thought that people who have MCI are at an increased risk of going on to develop Alzheimer's disease or another form of dementia. The Alzheimer's Society states that: 'In studies carried out in memory clinics, 10–15 per cent of people with MCI went on to develop dementia in each year that the research results were followed up. In community studies and clinical trials the rates are about half this level, but MCI still represents a significantly increased level of risk.'

However, many people with MCI improve or remain stable and do not develop dementia.

There are other 'lifestyle factors' that may increase the risk of developing dementia. These are covered extensively in my book *The Essential Guide to Avoiding Dementia* and are also described in chapter 9.

WHAT CAN I EXPECT?

Dementia progresses differently in different people but it is a progressive disease: the symptoms will become worse over time. There is no known cure.

The progression and outcome of dementia vary from person to person, but are largely determined by the type of dementia and which area of the brain is affected. The popular press usually emphasises the loss of short-term memory, but, although this is a classic symptom, it may not be the first sign that arouses anxiety in those developing dementia or their family. This emphasis on short-term memory may mean that people do not realise that other signs and symptoms may be more important in terms of indicating cognitive decline.

For convenience doctors sometimes talk about the 'stages' of dementia. This is a bit misleading as dementia does not progress in a standard way, but varies with each individual. Here is one view of the generally accepted stages of dementia:

Early dementia – In so-called 'early dementia', there are clear-cut deficits on careful clinical interview. For example, there might be difficulty performing complex tasks, such as handling finances, or travelling. Denial is common. There may be withdrawal from challenging situations. Someone with early dementia might be able to live independently – perhaps with assistance from family or caregivers.

Moderate dementia – People with 'moderate dementia' cannot survive alone without some assistance. They will be unable to recall major relevant aspects of their current lives, such as an address or telephone number of many years, or the names of grandchildren. There will be some disorientation as to the date, day of the week, season, or to place. They will probably require little assistance with toileting, eating, or dressing, but may need help choosing appropriate clothing. They generally live at home with live-in family members or other home support.

Moderately severe dementia – In 'moderately severe dementia', sufferers may occasionally forget the name of their spouse. They will be largely unaware of recent experiences and events in their lives. They will require assistance with basic activities of daily living ('ADLs') and they may be incontinent of urine. Behavioural and psychological symptoms of dementia ('BPSD' – see page 130) are common, such as delusions, repetitive behaviours and agitation. At this stage they may need to live in a residential care home.

Severe dementia – In reaching this stage, sufferers will have lost their verbal abilities – that is, their ability to use words. They will also have lost their ability to walk. They will be doubly incontinent and need assistance with feeding.

In fact everyone differs in the way their dementia progresses. Some people may lose the ability to speak in coherent sentences early on and this may be the prompt which causes them (or relatives on their behalf) to seek diagnosis. Loss of this ability may result in long pauses between words, or it may cause increasing silences and refusal to engage in normal social conversation. On the other hand, the person with dementia may continue to speak fluently for a long time but their sentences become confused and muddled and they may seem incoherent to those trying to talk to them.

Sometimes the ability to write is lost early on, although coherent speech is retained. Some people may notice that they are no longer able to sign their name. Interestingly, the ability to read (although not necessarily with comprehension) is often retained for many years after the onset of dementia.

Increasing inability to follow a sequence when performing common activities may be one of the first signs that there is something wrong. The person with dementia may find it difficult to put their clothes on in the right order, or to make a cup of tea, or to follow a recipe. These are actions we all perform for years almost automatically and so when this ability is lost it generally causes great consternation, prompting people to visit their doctor to seek a diagnosis.

The first indication that there was anything wrong was when my wife found herself in a muddle when cooking. She had always been a great baker of cakes, but suddenly it seemed she couldn't understand the recipe and there were several 'disasters' which ended with her in tears before I persuaded her to see the doctor. To be honest, I thought it might be something wrong with her sight so the diagnosis was a bit of a shock.

In common with the loss of ability to follow a sequence, loss of orientation may also alert family and friends that all is not well. Sometimes one of the first signs is 'getting lost' in a familiar environment or forgetting a commonly used route, such as the way to the local shops. In some cases, lack of orientation can be one of the biggest problems: the person with developing dementia can still hold conversations, carry out common tasks and continue to read and write, but they have difficulty finding their way about.

My wife started accusing me of hitting the ball in the wrong direction when we played a game of golf. I didn't realise what she meant at first but within quite a short time I found no one would play with me because I had no idea which way to face when playing. Not long after that I turned the wrong way when leaving the pub one night to walk home and if a friend had not chased after me I would have got hopelessly lost, even though I only lived half a mile away.

Initially the person with dementia is able to cope with normal activities provided they are not over-stressed. Difficulties may happen only occasionally and may be written off by family and friends as the natural 'slowing down' of increasing age. Lapses of memory may be covered up or go unnoticed; difficulties with following a television programme or the plot of a film passed off as due to tiredness. Practical problems with following a sequence of actions (dressing or following a recipe) can initially be overcome by taking more time or by preparation such as laying clothes out the night before. With help and regular support and care, the person with dementia can have a good quality of life, usually for some years.

The disease will progress over time (usually a few years) and there is no known cure. Medication can sometimes stabilise

people for a while but (for reasons which are not completely understood) the medication becomes less effective and people with
dementia will find that their capabilities deteriorate and their
ability to manage life independently disappears. As a general
rule, long-term residential care or intensive home support will
be needed eventually.

The effects of different causes early on

**Although the symptoms of dementia are often similar, the
early physical effects of various dementias on the brain and
the body are different.**

Medical science has discovered how the disease manifests in the
brain, but there is still a lack of knowledge about cause and effect.

In **Alzheimer's disease**, the two most common features are
plaques and tangles in the brain. These were first described by
Alois Alzheimer, after whom the disease was named. Plaques are
small clumps of a protein known as beta-amyloid, which usually
exists in the brain in a soluble form. With Alzheimer's disease the
amyloid clumps together into solid deposits known as **plaques**.
This disrupts the normal workings of the brain.

During the course of the disease, **tangles**, which look like dark
shapes, develop within the cells of the brain. They are made up
of a protein known as Tau. In a normal brain, Tau forms rope-like
structures that guide chemical messages and brain nutrients
down the axon (the long tail) of the cell to send messages on to
other cells. With Alzheimer's disease an abnormal form of Tau
accumulates that tangles up the rope-like structures. This causes
brain cells to die from lack of nutrients. Patients with Alzheimer's
also have a deficiency in the levels of some neurotransmitters – vital brain chemicals involved with the transmission of
messages. Eventually the brain begins to atrophy. Alzheimer's
disease tends to progress steadily with a slow decline in abilities.

However, some elderly people have many of these plaques and tangles in their brain but they do not display signs of dementia, so this is not the whole story.

Vascular dementia develops where problems with blood circulation result in parts of the brain not receiving enough blood and oxygen. We know that this can cause small areas of the brain to 'die'. Although the human brain can compensate for this (as evidenced by the number of people who recover function after a stroke), if enough areas are damaged so that they can no longer function, the ability to carry out everyday tasks and to learn anything new will be lost. In vascular dementia, the progress of the disease is often 'stepped'. Any new incident (such as a tiny stroke) will cause an abrupt decline in abilities, followed by a period of stability until the next incident.

At the time of writing, medical opinion is changing. The thinking is that even with plaques and tangles present in the brain, Alzheimer's disease is unlikely to develop without some precipitating factor – most probably a small stroke. This may be small enough to go unnoticed initially, but the disease progresses. For this reason, many doctors now often diagnose 'mixed dementia' rather than specifying vascular dementia or Alzheimer's disease.

In **dementia with Lewy bodies**, abnormal structures, known as Lewy bodies, develop inside the brain. These are tiny, spherical protein deposits found in nerve cells. Their presence in the brain disrupts its normal functioning, interrupting the action of important chemical messengers, including acetylcholine and dopamine. Researchers have yet to understand fully why Lewy bodies occur in the brain and how they cause damage. Lewy bodies are also found in the brains of people with Parkinson's disease, a progressive neurological disease that affects movement. People who have dementia with Lewy bodies may experience detailed and convincing visual hallucinations (seeing things that are not there), often of people or animals. They are also inclined to fall asleep very easily by day, and have restless, disturbed nights with confusion, nightmares and hallucinations. They may have stiff movements and tremors, faint or fall over and their abilities are likely to fluctuate daily or even hourly.

In **fronto-temporal dementia**, the frontal and temporal lobes of the brain begin to shrink. Unlike other types of dementia, fronto-temporal dementia usually develops in people who are under 65. It is much rarer than other types of dementia. People with fronto-temporal dementia often find that their memory is not affected so early in the disease as with other forms of dementia. Instead, speech may be affected and the social inhibitions that help us to behave in a considerate manner to others may be lost.

Can dementia be treated?

The different types of dementia may cause different symptoms at first but all of them are progressive. At present there is no cure and only limited treatment for some types.

All bodily functions rely upon the brain to work and as the brain becomes less and less able to function, so the person with a dementing illness will become less and less able to carry out the functions of everyday living. Eventually a person with dementia will become unable to walk, to swallow, even to breathe. In actual fact, most people die of an infection or some other illness before this happens.

Medical treatment can help some people with dementia but it cannot cure dementia or stop its progress.

Treatment (where available) varies with different types of dementia and this is one reason why early diagnosis is so important. Another reason is that, as with any progressive terminal illness, knowledge of the future allows people to make plans and indicate their wishes while they are still able to do so.

Drugs that may slow dementia's progress down

In Alzheimer's disease

Medication can improve symptoms, or temporarily slow down the progression of the disease in some people.

The key drugs used in cases of Alzheimer's disease are cholinesterase inhibitors and N-Methyl-D-aspartate (NMDA) receptor antagonists, which work in different ways. Cholinesterase inhibitors include donepezil hydrochloride (which you may know as 'Aricept'), rivastigmine (Exelon) and galantamine (Reminyl). The NMDA receptor antagonist is memantine (Ebixa).

Cholinesterase inhibitors do not work for everyone. Between 40 and 70 per cent of people with Alzheimer's disease benefit from cholinesterase inhibitor treatment but symptoms may improve only temporarily, for between six months and a couple of years in most cases. However, new research has indicated that even people with severe Alzheimer's disease may benefit from their use. People taking the drugs have experienced improvements in motivation, anxiety levels and confidence, as well as increased ability to deal with the tasks of daily living, and improved memory and thinking ability. Some people have claimed that the effect is 'like a miracle', while others notice no benefit. Identifying who will benefit can be difficult.

Memantine is licensed for the treatment of moderate-to-severe Alzheimer's disease. It can temporarily slow down the progression of symptoms, including loss of everyday functions, in people in the middle and later stages of the disease. There is evidence that memantine may also help with symptoms such as aggression and agitation.

In vascular dementia

Trials examining **cholinesterase inhibitors** for the treatment of **vascular dementia** indicate that the benefits for this type of dementia are very modest, except in individuals with a combination of both Alzheimer's disease and vascular dementia. Treatment for vascular dementia is usually concentrated on preventing further vascular problems and may include medication for stroke, high blood pressure, diabetes and heart problems.

In dementia with Lewy bodies

There is some evidence that the medications used for Alzheimer's disease are also effective for those who have **dementia with Lewy bodies.** People who are experiencing symptoms such as rigidity and stiffness may benefit from drugs used to treat Parkinson's disease, although these can make hallucinations and confusion worse. For people with dementia with Lewy bodies, neuroleptics (strong tranquillisers usually given to people with severe mental health problems) may be particularly dangerous.

In fronto-temporal dementia

The drugs used for treatment of Alzheimer's disease do not work for **fronto-temporal dementia** and indeed may make symptoms worse. Treatment is based around support and therapy (such as speech and language therapy).

WHAT ELSE CAN I DO?

There are lots of ways for people with dementia and their carers to help themselves – this book is one source of help.

Much of the treatment for dementia is centred around support for both people with dementia and their carers. Community psychiatric nurses, speech and language therapists, occupational therapists and dementia support workers can all get involved and show people with dementia how to manage their declining abilities. Carers, for example, can be taught strategies to manage challenging behaviour in those they care for.

People with dementia and those caring for them will need

help to apply for relevant financial help and support, aids and appliances to help with daily living, and help to find suitable day-care facilities, respite care and long-term residential care as required. There is robust evidence to show that good support at home can delay the need for long-term residential care. The Alzheimer's Society is an excellent source of help and support and, in some areas, community mental health teams work with Alzheimer Society Dementia Support workers and Dementia Advisers to provide ongoing support to those who have been diagnosed with any form of dementia and to those who care for them.

Whatever else you do, read this book either in detail or just the highlights, and plan ahead. Denial does not help anyone and it stands in the way of seeking help.

Chapter 2

Build a team

When dementia takes hold you need outside support because, as people get worse, they cannot be left alone for any length of time and the carer needs to share the burden with others.

Why do you need a support team? When it comes to dementia you cannot 'go it alone'. It doesn't matter whether you are independent and used to managing your own affairs, that you're 'not a sociable person' or are used to 'keeping yourselves to yourselves'. You as a couple (carer and person with dementia) may pride yourselves on one, any, or all of these virtues, but it is important once dementia strikes that you re-think your attitudes.

People who have dementia cannot manage alone except for a very short time. Because they have problems with their memory sequencing, they may think – and they may assure you – that they can manage very well. This is because they have managed in the past and are remembering those times. As their memory and cognitive function are no longer working properly, they forget all the occasions when things haven't gone so well.

If you are caring for a parent who lives alone it may be very tempting to believe them when they say they can manage. It will not be true. If you are caring for a spouse or partner, it will be more obvious that they are not managing – but it may nevertheless take you a while to realise this.

Couples who live together tend to support each other and sometimes increase that level of support without even realising they are doing so. It can be helpful to take a few moments to consider your life together now and how it was 10 years ago. Did your spouse/partner rely on you this much back then? If you are giving more support now (however subtly that level of support has increased) and if this is not due solely to physical disability, then their cognitive abilities have changed.

A person who has dementia can NOT live alone successfully, and in a perfect world we would never expect them to do so. 'Care packages' that involve carers calling in once, twice or even three times a day to help someone living alone are only a stop-gap measure. Very good carers who take pride in their work and genuinely care about their clients can make a difference, but they cannot replace the constant watchful presence that is required in all cases except the very early stages of dementia. Sometimes, however, this kind of care is the only and right option at the time and in this case it is important to get the very best care package that you can for as long as it is possible to manage this way.

On the other hand, spouses and partners who live with someone who has dementia are put under constant stress as they try to look after them. Living with another person – even when they are in good health – requires constant compromise as we adjust our habits, actions and conversation in the interests of 'rubbing along together'. Over many years these actions and adjustments become habitual, but they still remain. The most important thing to remember and take note of is that in any social situation all persons are involved in this constant compromise. Of course we can recognise that most partnerships are unequal and that one partner may make more adjustments than the other. Usually the person who makes more adjustments to the will of another does this willingly. Nevertheless, living with someone involves a constant daily compromise between pleasing ourselves and pleasing another. But people who have dementia gradually lose their ability to see another person's point of view – they lose their ability to empathise, to understand the everyday compromises that kept the partnership going. The partner who is the carer is left making all the compromises – possibly without even the satisfaction of a shared sense of humour or of togetherness – and certainly without the feelings of support they may have once had from their partner.

This is a burden that no one, however loving and dedicated, should carry alone.

If you are a carer in this situation, what can you do? You can build a team to help you.

WHO WILL BE ON YOUR TEAM?

Your support team can consist of anyone who is prepared to give time and help to you and the person you are caring for: family, friends, neighbours, professional carers, staff in a day centre and support workers from organisations such as the Alzheimer's Society can all be included.

Ask the family

It may be difficult to imagine family members as part of a support 'team' but most of us already rely on our family in many situations. There are many benefits to having members of the family as part of the team. The person you are caring for already knows them and feels comfortable with them. He/she will be used to their company and to their helping hand in some situations. Family members know the person with dementia from before the illness was diagnosed and these shared memories can be very important – as can the ability of family members to see beyond the dementia to the personality and character of the person they knew.

Elderly parents are often reluctant to ask their children for help. In my work I frequently meet people who tell me that their children are 'too busy' or 'lead such full lives' that they cannot ask them for any more of their time. This is a great pity and I would urge anyone who feels like that to think again. As you build your team, you will find that the amount of time and effort you ask from each helper is actually relatively small. Whilst it is true that adult children with families of their own may be very busy, most will be glad to help out – perhaps bearing in mind that the opportunity for these acts of kindness will not always be there.

Other family members such as brothers and sisters, cousins, nephews and nieces, if they have always been close and regular visitors, can play a valuable part in the team.

Tell family members about the diagnosis and ask your family to help.

Ask friends

Many people withdraw from society when dementia enters their lives. As explained in the section on Lifestyle (chapter 9), this is a bad thing in itself. However, for many people it becomes a big effort to keep their social life going. They may fear that friends are becoming less involved and withdrawing from their social circle. Many people think that dementia carries a 'stigma', which reduces their social circle and the number of people who might otherwise act as a support network.

The fact is that true friends do not feel this way. Friends care about those whom they have chosen as friends. Even casual acquaintances are often willing to help. The problem seems to be one of understanding. Good friends who want to help need to be kept in the loop so that they can understand what effect dementia has and how they can continue to be good friends and to offer their support as required. Ask your friends to help according to their ability.

I thought my friends Pam and Roger had become rather stand-offish. Pam always seemed in a hurry and although she seemed glad when I called she often did not invite me in as she had done in the past. If I asked after Roger she usually said that he was busy 'in the garden' or that he was still in bed (which I thought seemed very odd). It was only one day when I found her in tears that it all came out. Roger had Alzheimer's disease and she had been trying to keep it hidden. She seemed to be ashamed of the fact and felt embarrassed at allowing me to see Roger. Actually because it was quite a few months since I had seen him I thought Roger had changed a lot and was very confused and he didn't seem to know me. I stayed talking with him for half an hour that day and by the end of the visit he was actually talking much more sensibly and seemed more like the Roger I knew. I asked Pam if I could come again the next day and now I call round two or three times a week and often go for a walk with Roger or pop into the pub for a quick drink with him. It seems a small thing to do as we have always been friends.

Ask neighbours and casual acquaintances

While we generally hope to get along with our neighbours, most of us would balk at the idea of asking them to do anything more onerous than perhaps taking in a parcel if we are out. But your neighbours will be familiar to the person with dementia – he or she may forget their names but is still likely to know that the neighbour is someone familiar. It may be your neighbour who spots the person with dementia outside looking lost. It is likely to be your neighbour who notices the day the person with dementia misplaces his/her key and cannot get into the house.

Your neighbours often know quite a lot about your life and most people want to be good neighbours. If you explain the situation to your neighbours and help them to understand dementia they can be a tower of strength.

> *My husband wandered out of the front door one day while my back was turned and if it hadn't been for my neighbour spotting him I wouldn't have known in which direction he had gone.*

Tell your neighbours about the person with dementia and ask them to help you.

Use professional carers

You may decide early in the illness to employ professional carers, either to help with tasks you find difficult (including giving personal care) or to look after the person with dementia so that you can have time to yourself to carry out essential tasks or to go shopping or visit the hairdressers or meet the bank manager – any one of a hundred occasions when you do not want to be distracted. (Remember that you may be entitled to some help with care costs (see page 181).)

Some people do not want to employ a professional carer until they absolutely have to, either because they do not want to introduce a stranger into the household or because they feel guilty at 'not managing' everything themselves. Others prefer to pay someone to help with certain tasks from the diagnosis onwards. One advantage of doing this is that the person with dementia will have time to get to know them and to trust them. Also, as the main carer, you will also have time to decide whether they fit on your team and whether you can trust them to fulfil whatever duties you wish to give them. Remember that dementia is progressive and that you may need help at a later stage with things that are easy to manage earlier on. Agency care can be increased as and when you need it, but doing this is easier if you have built up a relationship with the care agency and its staff.

One other aspect of using professional carers is the fact that in such a case no one is doing you a favour. You pay for the care you want and you can expect the standard of care you pay for. You don't have to feel grateful to the carer, although of course you may do so and if you feel the standard falls short, you can say so and, if necessary, try an alternative agency.

Remember, the carers who staff a day centre are professional carers, specifically trained and selected because they enjoy working with people who have dementia. They will have experience and skill and can become part of your support team. If you are lucky enough to have contact with a local dementia adviser or support worker from an organisation such as the Alzheimer's Society, this person too will be a valuable part of your team. You can turn to them for advice and information at any time that you need to.

CHOOSING AND BUILDING YOUR TEAM

It is important to make a plan so that you know exactly what you do need rather than letting yourself feel overwhelmed. What are the gaps that the person with dementia once filled? What do you find difficult?

Building your support team is one of the most important things you can do in coping with dementia. Who you choose for your team depends upon many factors. You need people who can help you to do the things you cannot do or which you find difficult. You need people who are willing to help the person with dementia do the things that he/she can no longer manage alone. The person you are caring for may have played an important part in the activities of your everyday life. For example, he or she may have been good at DIY and kept the home ticking over by changing plugs, putting up shelves or painting and decorating. Or perhaps he/she did the cooking, housework or laundry. Someone will have to take over these duties gradually. That someone may be you or you may decide to find someone who can do these things for you . You also need people to give you some respite – that is, time off from your caring duties

Of course, everyone's needs are different. You will have to think ahead. Some people find personal care for a partner or parent no trouble – they consider it part of a loving relationship. Others find that providing this type of care interferes with their established relationship. Some people enjoy finding simple pastimes or non-challenging activities for the person with dementia to do – others find this extremely tedious. Some carers find outings and social occasions with the person who has dementia enjoyable. Others find them embarrassing or frustrating. There is no need to feel guilty or force yourself to do things that may lead you to be short tempered and less patient with the person you care for.

A calm and patient carer makes for a calm and contented person with dementia. You need to help yourself as well as the one you are caring for.

Generally most people find that, if they cannot cope with personal care, then paying for a professional carer from a reputable agency is the best option. Often, although initially resistant, the person with dementia prefers a professional to help with intimate care.

Friends, relatives and neighbours are the best option if you want to arrange for someone to take part in leisure activities and pastimes with the person with dementia, although some professional carers from an agency will also do this.

Kind neighbours and friends may carry out DIY, maintenance or gardening tasks, but you may prefer to find a local handyman or gardening service you can call on when needed. It is hard to keep chasing a busy neighbour up about a task without feeling you might be nagging.

If you need help with housework, cleaning and laundry, you can pay for a cleaning service. Some professional caring agencies also include light housework among their carer's duties.

If you can afford to, you can pay for help with cooking, but it may be easier to learn to do this yourself and there are so many convenience foods available these days that most people can eat quite well even if they are not accomplished cooks. (See the tips on nutrition in chapter 9 and remember that people with dementia need nutrient-rich foods). Alternatively, you might make a meals delivery service part of your team.

For outings, friends and family are probably the best people to call on.

People who, take the person with dementia out, who carry out activities with them or even just sit and keep them company, are all providers of respite care – they enable the main carer to have some time off. Day centres and residential respite care in a care home also allow for longer periods of respite, when the carer knows that he/she will have a whole day, several days, or even a week's break from the constant caring duties. There is further discussion of respite options in chapter 12 (see page 202).

Inviting people to join your team

People may want to help but only feel able to join your team if you ask them to do something specific. Then they will know what you need and whether they can be relied on to do it.

You may think that asking people to be on your team is a daunting task. It may seem to you as if no one would want to take on the tasks you need help with. In fact, most people (once they understand what the diagnosis of dementia means to you) will be pleased to help. You don't have to tell them they are joining your team in so many words. You can simply ask them to help.

When you do ask for help be very specific. If you say, 'As you know. John has dementia and it would really be kind if you could lend me a hand with him now and again,' people will probably smile and say, 'Of course – just give me a call.' This means that you have to stiffen your resolve later to ask the favour again. It is best at the outset to say something like, 'It would be lovely if you could come and sit with John on Thursday afternoons,' so that everybody is clear about what is needed.

First think about what sort of help you need. Try to think ahead a bit, because dementia is a progressive condition. Just because John can find his way down to the paper shop each morning and buy a paper and find his way home again now, doesn't mean that he will always be able to do this. Of course, dementia develops differently in each individual so planning is not easy. If you don't feel confident about how the progression might go, you can talk to a dementia support worker about this. The clues are often there. Someone who has lost his/her way once will be liable to do this again, although maybe not every day. Someone who has difficulty signing his/her name will probably lose the ability to write quite soon, although he/she may be able to carry out many other activities of everyday living.

Once you have an idea of where you need help, decide who might be best placed to offer help in that area and then ASK THEM. A specific request is more likely to get a straightforward answer, whether positive or negative.

Here are some examples of straightforward specific requests:

'John is likely to get confused and lose his way these days. Would you be able just to walk down to the paper shop with him in the mornings to keep him company in case he gets confused?'

'Your father would love to go to the pub for a drink occasionally.

Could you call round once a week and take him?'

'Can you take your mother shopping on Saturday to buy some new underwear?'

'Thank you for offering to help. I know Fred would like to keep up his outings to the football club. Would you be able to call round and go there with him on Mondays?'

'Mollie would like to keep going to church on Sundays and in the past I've been happy to take her and pick her up. But she sometimes gets confused now when she is there on her own. As you go to the same church, could she go with you and sit with you during the service? I'd be happy to take and collect you both in the car.'

With requests like this you are asking for only one specific piece of help and whoever you ask knows what is expected of them. If you are clever and think about the members of your team, you will find you are only asking people to do what they are already doing. You are just making the arrangement more clear cut. If your husband has always gone to the football club with the neighbour two doors down and you ask for this arrangement to continue, your neighbour is unlikely to feel awkward about it. On the other hand, because you have made a specific request he/she will not be tempted to allow the regular outing to drop because 'Fred isn't up to it any more', until that genuinely is the case.

Potential team members may need to know more about dementia. They may be concerned it makes sufferers violent, though this is rarely the case. Recommend they visit the websites listed at the end of this book, or print off spreadsheets from the Alzheimer's Society for them.

If some of your 'team' ask for more information about dementia, try to make sure that they can access it. You can give them the information you know yourself but some people prefer to read the facts at their leisure so that they can take them in at their own pace. The factsheets issued by the Alzheimer's Society (www.alzheimers.org.uk) are an excellent source of authoritative information and they can be downloaded from the Society's website or ordered from them by phone. You can also tell your team about any carers' information courses that are being run locally, or lend them suitable books. Your dementia support worker, if you have one, will be pleased to explain about dementia to members of your team. Try not to listen to spurious media information such as, 'It said in the Daily X today that there is a pill to cure dementia' and be prepared to gently discourage any well-meant attempts to 'put you right' as a result of this.

> *My husband's friend was very kind and helpful at first but then he started telling me that he had read on the web that 'people with Alzheimer's are frightened of water'. I was having difficulty in getting Peter to shower sometimes but this seemed to be more because he couldn't get himself going in the mornings. I got very confused when his friend started saying this but I noticed that once in the shower Peter really enjoyed his wash. I changed our routine so that he showered before bed, which was when he was less sluggish and this worked quite well.*

What to do if someone says no

Supposing someone refuses your request for their help? It may be because they are frightened and worried. Many people believe that those with dementia 'become violent' and there is certainly a tendency for the general public to associate the confusion and frustration felt by someone with dementia with violence. If this is the case, helping the worried person to understand more about dementia will make a difference – again use the sources of help and information detailed above. Although people with dementia may become agitated and even hit out if put in a really difficult situation, most retain their sense of what is acceptable public behaviour and do not do this. (See also the section on 'challenging behaviour' on page 56.) In this situation it may be good to ask someone like a nurse or a dementia adviser or support worker to explain the facts to your potential helper.

Sometimes people may feel unable to help because they are afraid of being put under an obligation or of agreeing to an arrangement they may not be able to keep. It is worth giving your helper a get-out clause, when making your specific request for help. For example:

'Of course, I know you sometimes don't go to church if the weather is very bad and naturally I wouldn't expect you to put yourself out in that case.'

'I know the time may come when it will be too difficult to take Fred to the club and when you feel that time has come I will quite understand.'

You need to be able to rely on your team members – if people let you down you will know you have to find someone else.

At least if someone refuses to help, you will know where you stand. It is more difficult to manage the people who agree to help and then do not turn up when expected or make spurious excuses to avoid a regular arrangement. For someone with dementia, any variation in routine is likely to arouse anxiety and they will not be able to understand sudden changes in arrangements. No matter how carefully you explain that 'Jim telephoned to say that he couldn't come to the pub with you today because he has to look after the children,' the person you are caring for may react by behaving awkwardly. For you, the carer, an unreliable team member is worse than none at all.

Michael's sister said she would come to spend the afternoon with him while I saw a couple of my friends for coffee and a shopping trip. But she just didn't turn up. Michael had seen me getting ready and we both waited and waited but she didn't even phone to say she couldn't come. We both had a very upsetting day.

In a case like this the best thing is to assume the person concerned will not fit on your team and to try to look for someone to replace them.

The process of building your team and of planning how you might get regular relief from care may seem a major and complicated task and even unnecessary, particularly if you are reading this chapter shortly after an early diagnosis. However, you should take advantage of the fact that you have time to plan and organise: building your team will make your life (and the life of the person with dementia) more tolerable and even enjoyable in the long run.

Chapter 3

Understanding the health and social care system

One of the most difficult things to come to terms with after a diagnosis of dementia is the feeling that your life is no longer your own. This chapter will help you, as a carer, to understand the role of some of the people you may meet, such as health professionals, social-care professionals and support professionals, and people working for voluntary organisations. I will explain the meaning of care plans and support plans and will also give you help to find your way through the maze of hospital visits, respite care and support organisations.

The path to diagnosis is not straightforward; there are thought to be large numbers of people who have dementia but their illness has yet to be diagnosed. Perhaps you have bought this book because you are worried that someone you know has dementia and you are hoping to find ways to cope with this? It may be, on the other hand that this book has come into your hands as a result of a diagnosis and you are hoping that you will find in here the answers to the many questions in your mind. It may even be that you have been supporting someone with a diagnosis of dementia for some time but that you feel the need of a reference to guide you.

Getting a diagnosis can take time. There are other causes of memory problems to rule out and getting someone with

memory problems to appreciate they need help can be challenging.

GETTING A DIAGNOSIS

Let us first consider the question of getting a diagnosis. Perhaps you have been worried for some time about someone whom you are close to and you think that they may have dementia. There are many supposedly helpful leaflets and advertisements in the media suggesting what you should do if you are 'worried about your memory', but if you care for someone with memory problems you may well have discovered that these are unhelpful. The fact is that most people who have the beginnings of dementia are not worried about their memory. One of the many features of dementia is a lack of insight into the problems the illness is causing. Most people with dementia do not think that they have a problem. If someone has cognitive problems, they may not realise that they do because their powers of reasoning are impaired. It is as simple as that.

Doctors and nurses can compound this in the eyes of the carer because there is a drive these days towards transparency and collective decision making in healthcare. Of course it is quite correct that healthcare professionals should not talk about people behind their backs and they should be open and 'up front' in discussing health problems, but this can be most unhelpful in the case of dementia. When the doctor asks someone with dementia if he/she is having any problems with memory or with everyday activities, the patient is likely to say that he/she does not have any problems. The carer is left feeling that the doctor does not understand what is happening, particularly if the doctor refuses to meet with the carer privately in the interests of 'confidentiality'.

If you are worried that someone close to you has cognitive problems, you have probably already discovered that there is little to be gained by pointing this out to them. A few people who have a close and trusting relationship can accept their relative or partner's word and act upon it, but the majority of people with cognitive problems are unable to accept that there is anything wrong. Indeed, many people in the early stages of dementia may get quite annoyed if errors and mistakes are pointed out to them; they may become angry and begin to accuse those nearest to them of 'plotting' against them or 'ganging up' on them or of deliberately hiding items or stealing from them.

If you are worried that you have cognitive problems, then you should make an appointment to discuss this with your doctor. If you are worried that someone else has a problem, the situation is more difficult. You may be able to persuade them to see their doctor if they trust you and can accept that there seems to be a problem. It is also worth remembering that memory problems can be the result of things other than dementia. For example, some prescription drugs can affect memory; thyroid problems can make people tired and slow; a severe vitamin shortage can affect cognition (is the sufferer eating properly?) and a urinary-tract infection (see chapter 10, page 167) can cause dementia-like symptoms. The only way to find out the cause of the problem is to be examined by a doctor.

If you cannot persuade the person you care about to consult his/her doctor, it can be very difficult. You can try writing to their GP and telling them your worries. Then at least those concerns will be on file, giving the doctor the opportunity to check the person's memory when he/she next goes along to see the doctor about something unrelated. It is unlikely that the GP will discuss your worries with you for reasons of patient confidentiality. If the person you care for attends hospital as an inpatient, any signs of dementia will probably be picked up then and followed up.

Generally the GP will run some tests to eliminate other causes for the symptoms and if these come back negative, a referral will probably be made to a consultant psychiatrist who specialises in the health of older people, to a geriatrician (a consultant who cares for older people) or sometimes to a neurologist. The referral process will differ according to your local health practice. In some areas patients may be seen by a community psychiatric nurse working in a team managed by a consultant psychiatrist.

It may take some time for a diagnosis to be made. You should not feel annoyed by this as it means that the doctors and mental-health specialists are taking care to ensure that the final diagnosis is correct. If you are worried in the meantime you can encourage the person you are caring for to take some simple self-help steps (see chapter 9, page 147 and also my book *The Essential Guide to Avoiding Dementia*).

If you are finally diagnosed with dementia you may be offered medication; you should certainly be offered support.

HEALTH PROFESSIONALS EXPLAINED

You and the person you are caring for may come into contact with many people and organisations after a diagnosis of dementia. It can be quite confusing knowing who to turn to in different situations and often different sources of support seem to overlap. It is good to get into the habit of noting down the names of those who contact you (ask for a business card) and perhaps keeping a separate file with appointment letters, notes, names and contact details and copies of any forms you may have to complete. In my work I am often amazed at the number of people who have given intimate details about their health and social condition to others but who do not remember who they spoke to or what organisation they represented.

Always ask for proof of identification when anyone contacts you or calls at your home, and keep a note of their name and of what follow-up they promised.

After a diagnosis of dementia people in the UK are generally kept under the care of the **local community mental health team**

(CMHT). The team comprises psychiatrists, psychologists, community psychiatric nurses (CPNs) and sometimes occupational therapists (OTs), speech and language therapists (SALTs), and support workers. Some teams also have a social liaison worker attached to them who is employed by social services. The health professional that the person with dementia sees regularly will differ according to where you live.

The service that encompasses access to all the professionals mentioned above is sometimes called the 'memory clinic'.

The person you care for may see a consultant psychiatrist regularly at first. This should not alarm you. These people are specialists in the mental health of older people and will have up-to-date knowledge about dementia. It is best if you accompany the person with dementia to their appointments as the consultant will need to ask you about symptoms and about any problems you are encountering. People with dementia often forget to mention relevant points to the doctor and, as I have said before, may not realise that they even have a problem.

If the person you care for has been diagnosed after a private consultation rather than within the NHS, you may not be referred to all the follow-up support available. Most people affected by dementia say that the support they receive is more important than the medical treatment so it is always worth enquiring about follow-up support if you are not automatically offered this.

Follow-up health support appointments will usually be with a member of the community mental health team. If the case is complex, then the person you care for may be referred to a community psychiatric nurse (CPN). Occasionally it may be the CPN who will give you the diagnosis under the direction of the consultant psychiatrist or gerontologist in charge of the team.

Sometimes after the diagnosis has been confirmed and treatment is proceeding, the person with dementia may be referred to a support worker from the CMHT who will be trained to monitor the situation and report back to the team if necessary.

Additional specific health support may be given by an occupational therapist, a speech therapist or a physiotherapist specialising in preventing falls.

As the disease progresses it may be important for you to receive help from an occupational therapist who has been trained to assess the abilities and the living area of the person with dementia and can recommend any aids to living (for example, hand rails or walking aids) which will help to maintain independence.

The speech and language therapists can be very helpful to carers by recommending better methods of communicating with those who are having speech difficulties. They are also experts in assessing the swallowing abilities of people who may have difficulties in this area; swallowing difficulties can often be experienced by someone who has dementia.

People who have difficulty with balance and who have frequent falls may be referred to a specialist 'falls team' who will assess what aids will help, recommend ways of managing balance and show carers the best way to help people who have fallen over to get back on their feet.

Sometimes people with dementia are referred to a memory clinic. This is simply the name for a service which encompasses access to all the professionals mentioned above.

Health problems which are not dementia related will continue to be dealt with by the GP, or, where necessary, by access services which relate to individual conditions such as a Diabetic nurse, or an asthma clinic.

THE SOCIAL SUPPORT TEAM EXPLAINED

Social workers help with non-health related problems and are part of the adult social care team. They offer care and support for adults who need extra help to manage their lives and be as independent as possible – including people with dementia and their carers.

Adult social care includes an assessment of needs – for both the person with dementia and the carer – and provision of services or provision of funding to allow the purchase of care and support. These services include extra care at home, day services, provision of aids and adaptations, personal budgets and residential care. Not everyone is eligible to receive help free, but everyone is entitled to a free care-needs assessment to enable them to work out what help they do need.

Social workers have different titles and job descriptions, but they should all carry identification and ask your permission to offer their services.

Some people can become quite worried if a suggestion is made that they may be referred to the social care team, but it is worth accepting this help if it is offered. You can consider whether the social workers will be part of your 'team' (see chapter 2).

VOLUNTARY AND OTHER SUPPORT ORGANISATIONS

Support is given by a number of mostly voluntary organisations and availability varies in different areas.

You may be put in contact with one or more voluntary organisations as a result of the diagnosis of dementia. In this regard, the most obvious voluntary organisation that comes to mind is the Alzheimer's Society whose workers support people with any form of dementia, not just Alzheimer's disease (see chapter 1 – What is dementia?). In many areas of the country, NHS healthcare professionals will refer people who have been diagnosed with dementia and their carers to the Alzheimer's Society as a matter of routine. However, there are areas where this does not happen and in this case it is a simple matter to contact a support worker from the Society independently. You can find contact details in your area on the Alzheimer's Society website (www.alzheimers. org.uk). Support workers from the Alzheimer's Society will be able to help you with advice, information and support to manage caring in the best way possible. Homecare workers in some areas will visit your home and care for the person with dementia to allow the carer some 'time off' from caring duties. The Society also runs day centres which specialise in giving a safe environment for the person with dementia in which they can experience stimulating and attractive activities.

Support groups are run not just by the Alzheimer's Society but also by carers' support organisations in many areas. You may find these of great benefit. We all have times when our patience runs out or we find it difficult to cope and being able to voice our feelings in a safe and confidential environment can help. You can also often get tips from other carers who have been going through the same stresses as you are experiencing. You can find details of groups run for carers in your area on the Alzheimer's Society website or on the website of Carers UK (www.carersuk. or). Telephone contact numbers are listed in the reference section of this book.

Other voluntary organisations that give general support to older adults also often run support services for people diagnosed with dementia. If you are not directed to these as a matter of course, then you can find out what is available in your area by consulting your local authority website, asking for information at the library or enquiring at your GP surgery. Some sources of support are listed in the reference section and more information is available on the website www.Adaptdementia.com.

Note: Citizens Advice Bureaux (CAB) are a very good resource if you need financial advice or advice about housing and social needs. Local CAB offices are listed on their website. Your local library is always a good source of information if you do not use the internet and need to contact voluntary organisations in your area.

CARE PLANS

A care plan is a written statement of how the person with dementia can best be cared for, and can be drawn up by health-care professionals or by social workers. You may have more than one care plan, each relating to different types of care.

Every health and support organisation should offer you a care plan. A care plan is written after an assessment has been done and is meant to set out what your care and support needs are or, in the case of health professionals, what your medical needs are. So there might be several different care plans which all refer to the same person but which differ according to the organisation drawing the care plan up.

For example, the care plan written by a social care worker might suggest a need for extra help in the house and detail how this is to be managed – perhaps by employing a care agency worker. The care plan of a dementia support worker might focus on the support needs you might have, such as a referral to a carers' support group, an application for benefits or help with organising a power of attorney (see page 182). The care plan drawn up by a residential care home would focus on the resident's needs, wishes and preferences in the matter of everyday care – for example, whether they like to be addressed formally or informally, whether they like a daily bath or a shower. The worker drawing up the care plan should discuss and agree it with the person with dementia and their carer. Care plans will change over time as the disease progresses.

Carers can have care plans, too. A social care worker might draw up a plan focused on your needs – perhaps including a referral to a carers' support group, help with organising lasting power of attorney or LPA (see chapter 11, page 182) or arranging respite care (see chapter 12, page 202).

The Essential Carer's Guide to Dementia

HOSPITAL APPOINTMENTS AND STAYS IN HOSPITAL

Out-patient departments

Generally people with dementia are able to understand when they have an appointment with a doctor at a hospital outpatients' department and they will be able to co-operate and take part in an examination or medical test as appropriate. However, they may not always be able to answer the doctor's questions and they may not find it easy to follow any instructions given to them. For this reason it is important that someone always accompanies them to an appointment.

It is also a good idea to try to arrange the appointment for a time when the person with dementia is less likely to be confused (some people are more confused very early in the morning or late in the afternoon, especially when darkness sets in early (see 'sundowning – chapter 4, page 61)). If possible, try to choose a time when they are not hungry or tired.

It is reasonable – and helpful – for the carer to explain to the doctor that the patient has a diagnosis of dementia, but if you feel that this will be difficult or embarrassing to do in front of the person you are caring for, then phone in advance to warn the doctor – or ask the receptionist to mention this to the doctor before your appointment. Although you should, of course, allow the person with dementia to answer any questions that they can and also ask any questions that they wish to, you should bear in mind that it is more important for their health that the doctor they are seeing gets the true picture. In this instance it may be important that you correct them (in a kind and tactful way) if they give incorrect answers about their health.

People with dementia can become agitated if they have to wait for a long period – this may be partly because they forget why they are in the waiting room at all. They may need regularly reminding of why they are there. Try not to let your own anxiety show and, as far as possible, keep a calm demeanour. If you have to leave the waiting room to walk about, for example, make sure the receptionist knows where you will be in case your name is called.

If the appointment is for a health problem other than memory it is worth making sure that the person with dementia knows this, because it may ensure that he/she is less anxious. Seeing the 'memory doctor' or waiting for a 'memory test' can be very stressful for someone with dementia.

In the accident and emergency (A&E) department

If the worst happens and the person you care for has a fall or an accident and the ambulance is called, he/she will be taken to the nearest hospital with an accident and emergency (A&E) unit and this is where he/she will wait to be assessed. Most A&E units now operate a 'triage' system. People arriving at the unit will be seen by a senior and specially trained nurse who will assess how quickly they need to be seen by a doctor. If you are with someone who has been taken to A&E you will find that the length of time you have to wait will depend on many things including the seriousness of any injury they may have, the number of other more serious cases awaiting attention, the time of day and the day of the week. Sunday night is still traditionally the worst day/time on which to have an accident requiring care in A&E. While waiting you should not allow the one you care for to eat or drink unless the nursing staff have told you that you may do so as this may interfere with any anaesthetic they may need. It is particularly important to check with the nursing staff if the person with dementia is also diabetic.

Waiting to be seen can be stressful for both you and the person with dementia. Hospitals differ in their level of care and efficiency but the most common complaint from those waiting is lack of information. Although the unit looks busy and is crowded with people in uniform of various kinds, it may seem a daunting task just to find out what is happening in your individual case, especially if the person you care for cannot be left.

If you are with someone with dementia they will need you to act for them. It is worth remembering that A&E departments have performance 'targets' that they are supposed to maintain in terms of waiting time for patients and treatment. You may not want to appear to be the one 'making a fuss' but persistence generally pays off in terms of getting attention. You should make sure that staff know that you are with someone who has dementia. You should be allowed to stay with them while they are examined if this will make them calmer and more co-operative. Don't be afraid to be assertive, but don't confuse assertive with aggressive. Most hospitals have very strong 'non-aggression' policies and they are rightly concerned about any form of aggression or violence shown to staff.

Some hospitals now have a ward where people are admitted temporarily. It may be called the 'medical assessment unit' or the 'short stay ward' and it is usually close to the A&E department. The person you are caring for may be admitted here if the results of tests and X-rays taken in A&E do not point to an instant diagnosis and hospital staff feel that they should not be sent home immediately. Again you should make sure that staff know that the person has dementia and ask if you can stay with them if possible. Medical assessment units are very busy and confusing – even for someone who is not cognitively impaired.

Staying in hospital

In general, a stay in hospital nearly always results in deterioration in cognitive ability for the person with dementia. For this reason you should avoid a hospital stay unless it is absolutely necessary. Naturally it is not a good idea to refuse an operation or hospital stay that is necessary for continued health and well-being or that will reduce pain. However, sometimes minor procedures can be done as a 'day case'. On other occasions, you might decide that, on balance, the small improvement to general health that an operation would bring does not outweigh the likely resulting deterioration in cognitive ability.

If the person you care for is admitted to the elderly care department (you may still think of it under the old term 'geriatric care') do not be alarmed. Times have changed and elderly care wards are now better staffed and better organised than they were in the past. Much of the basic 'hands-on' care of patients is now carried out by healthcare assistants (they may have another title – it varies from hospital to hospital). They have more time to spend with patients than the nurses do and most of them are well trained and enjoy working with elderly people. These are the staff who will help the person you care for get washed and dressed; they will make them comfortable, chat to them and if necessary help them at meal times. It is worth you getting to know them. You will also find that careful records are kept not only of medicines and treatment given but of individual care. For example, the care assistants will note that they have helped someone to shower or washed their hair and so on. Notes about this care are usually kept in a folder near the bed – you can read them when you visit and ask any questions about care and medication.

There will also usually be a leaflet or folder which gives details of the facilities available at the hospital for your cared-for and of any extra help that you need to provide – for example, in terms of taking away clothing and nightclothes to be washed and returned. It is worth trying to arrange for a member of the family to visit every day, not only to cheer up the person with dementia but also to keep a watchful eye on the level of care provided. If any assessment is to be made by a specialist, you can ask to be present and you should definitely talk to the doctor in charge of the case. The doctor's name will usually be displayed on a sign somewhere near the bed or on a ward plan available for all to see.

Elderly people, even if they are mentally alert, may still be in awe of the doctor and may not react quickly enough to ask relevant questions when they are examined or may not know what questions to ask. A person with dementia may not be able to answer questions correctly or at all. If you are not a relative but are the principal carer it is important to make this clear, especially if you have lasting power of attorney for health and welfare (see chapter 11, page 187) of the person you are caring for – otherwise you may not be given full information.

Many health authorities now have a system, variously named ('hospital passport' is one name in use), where the patient brings with him/her a previously prepared chart that states some personal history, some likes and dislikes, and important personal information. The Alzheimer's Society also produces a chart called 'This is Me', which you can fill out and take into hospital for the person with dementia. Ideally this should be kept with the medical charts at the end of the bed and consulted by the nursing and care staff. This is an excellent idea but does depend on the information being provided in the first place and whether it is kept up to date – and on the staff actually reading the document. This sort of chart is also useful if the person you are caring for has to go into a home for respite care or if he/she moves permanently into residential care. Update it regularly as the disease progresses.

Hospital schemes that include specialist dementia-trained staff

Hospitals are more aware of, and staff are more knowledgeable about, dementia these days. Many hospitals operate a special scheme that identifies patients with dementia and ensures that staff understand how to look after someone who is cognitively impaired. The schemes have various names in different hospitals. One well-known national one is the Butterfly Scheme, where hospitals offer patients and carers the opportunity to 'opt in' to the scheme. If you do so, a butterfly symbol is placed next to the patient's name in the ward lists and above their bed. Under the scheme, staff have been trained to respond positively and appropriately to people with dementia. They follow a special response plan, which includes important elements such as (taken from the Butterfly Scheme's notes):

- Reminding patients with dementia what is going on whenever a member of staff approaches them.
- Explaining procedures that are about to happen.
- Situating the bed in the most 'dementia friendly' place possible, which could be close to the nurses' station, or perhaps to the bathroom.
- Keeping the area beside the bed looking the same; making sure important possessions are available and accessible, always in the same place.
- Paying special attention to cleanliness and hydration (drinking enough water) – people with dementia may be unable to manage these things for themselves.
- Taking extra care when checking medical history with the carer.

Carers of people who have been opted into the Butterfly Scheme will be asked to fill in a special carer's sheet to give further information.

The Butterfly Scheme, and similar plans to give appropriate care to people with dementia or confusion, are an excellent idea. The implementation of these schemes varies from hospital to hospital and, as always, any scheme is only as good as the staff who put it into practice. The most important factor in helping to care for someone with dementia is time and in a busy hospital ward even well-intentioned and well-trained staff do not always have the time required. Where possible, do your best to stay with the person you care for, for as long as you can, and help hard-pressed staff by giving information and undertaking any caring tasks that you are able to.

What happens when it's time to leave the hospital?

The length of time someone spends in hospital obviously depends on how quickly they recover. It is unlikely that the person you care for will be allowed home until an assessment has been made of their home circumstances. If the hospital staff consider the person you care for to be vulnerable, they may ask the hospital social care team to get involved at this stage – even if they have not been so before.

As the carer, you can ask for an assessment of the person with dementia by the hospital social care team. In theory, a member of the team is always available during the day but it may not always be easy to arrange to talk to them. If you are worried about the person you care for coming home because you feel that you can no longer cope with the level of care they need, or because you feel you need extra help, you must make this clear to hospital staff at every opportunity. Sadly, there have been occasions reported where people with dementia are discharged from hospital and sent home without any extra support.

My mother-in-law lived with us and had to go into hospital for a hernia repair. Although I repeatedly told the staff that I would not be able to cope with her at home in the immediate aftermath, she was discharged back home after the procedure. She was confused and belligerent. She constantly clawed at the dressings over her wound and eventually it started to bleed. I called the ambulance and she was taken back to hospital, her wound was re-dressed and the doctor wanted to discharge her back home again. I told him I would not be able to cope and his response was 'What do you expect me to do – sit up all night watching her?' In the end this is what I had to do!

Hospital staff in charge of discharging patients are obliged to take the patient's wishes into account and it is very likely that someone with dementia will express a strong wish to return home – even though their carer feels unable to manage their care. People with dementia may not be able to understand the burden they are placing on their carer.

Help when you get back home

The hospital may suggest that the person you have been caring for can be discharged home with a suitable 'package of care'. This generally means trained professional carers who will come into the home up to three times a day to help with washing, dressing, managing the toilet and helping someone to eat. It may also include a plan for day care on one or more days each week to give you a break. Given this level of support you may feel able to manage, but don't be afraid of telling the hospital if you feel you won't be able to.

When someone with dementia is living alone an occupational therapy (OT) assessment of the home may be made to see if they can cope when they go home. If you are the chief carer for someone living alone and you have any doubts about their ability to manage, you should voice them to the OT team. If the person you care for is taken on a visit home for an assessment, try to be there too, as you may notice things that the OT team, however vigilant and well trained, may not – simply because you know the person and their home so well.

Re-ablement or intermediate care

The aim of 're-ablement' or 'intermediate care' (terminology differs in different areas) is to get people out of hospital and back home sooner than would otherwise be the case – ideal when the patient is keen to get back home. If, following an operation or admission after an accident, you and the person you care for could manage at home with just a little extra help to begin with, then it is possible that you might be eligible for help from the re-ablement or intermediate care team. This is available through social services, through the district nursing team or through direct referral from the hospital.

The team will be able to supply care assistants to help the person with dementia with simple everyday personal care, including meal preparation, up to three times a day for up to six weeks. If you feel this would be appropriate and it is not offered, make enquiries about it. Sometimes you may have to pay for this care. After the initial period of 're-ablement', you can pay for help from a care agency if you think you still need it. If you cannot afford to do this, you may be eligible for help from the social care team but the assessment of your financial situation and your needs may take some time. For this reason it is best to contact the social care team as soon as possible after hospital discharge. (Note that it cannot be done before because the community social care team will not get involved whilst a patient is under the care of the hospital social care team.)

Convalescence

An alternative to going straight home is for the person you care for to be admitted to a local community hospital or to a care or nursing home for a period of convalescence. You may have to be insistent to get this sort of care. Unfortunately beds in community hospitals are in high demand and a place in a care or nursing home may be available only if you are prepared to pay. However, do not be put off if you really feel that you will not be able to manage the person with dementia at home. Local authorities and social services have what is known as a 'duty of care' and they must make a proper assessment and offer adequate help. You may find that subtle pressure is put upon you by the hospital – they like to free up beds as soon as possible and are impatient with 'bed blockers'. They too have targets to meet. But your concern is with the safety and comfort of the person you care for.

When the person with dementia is finally discharged, all the relevant professionals should be informed by the hospital discharge team – these could include, for example, the district nursing team if appropriate, the carer's agency (if you use one), and social services. It's a good idea if you contact any vital services yourself, too, to make sure they've been informed. You could also try to insist that the person you care for is not discharged just before a weekend, because some of the support teams do not have full services available then. However, it is policy in most hospitals these days to discharge patients on any day of the week, so you may have no choice in the matter.

Following a stay in hospital, people with dementia are often initially more confused than before they were admitted. Sometimes they recover back to the cognitive level they were at before they went into hospital (short-term memory loss can actually be an advantage here as they may forget any trauma quickly), but this may take a little time and you will need to be patient and understanding. Often people with dementia do not recover well following a hospital stay and their cognitive abilities may deteriorate. It can help to be aware of this possibility.

Repeated hospital stays due to a series of infections or perhaps to constant falls may mean you need to re-think your care plans and perhaps consider long-term residential care.

Chapter 4

Difficulties and challenges

There are times when carers face particular difficulties and have to deal with what medical professionals often call 'challenging behaviour'. We each find different things 'challenging' and while one carer deals smoothly and without fuss with, say, problems of incontinence, but cannot cope with endless repetition, another blithely answers the same question asked countless times but gets upset by a refusal to eat or by drastic weight loss.

Many of the difficult behaviours that carers have to deal with are an enigma. For example, doctors and researchers do not know why some people with dementia become so much more unsettled around late afternoon and they have only a limited number of drugs and behavioural tactics to help carers cope with this. This chapter will help you try to work out why the person you care for is exhibiting difficult behaviour and suggests methods that you can use to cope. The behaviours I look at are the most common, but not everyone with dementia experiences all or indeed any of these:

- The inability to understand the meaning of time and distinguish between night and day (see page 56)
- Wandering and restlessness (see page 58)
- Incontinence (see page 62)
- Appetite and weight loss (see page 63)
- Aggression (see page 65)

- Loss of inhibition (see page 65)
- Being clinging and demanding (see page 67).

What challenges one person may not be problematic for another, but caring during the day followed by broken nights can make anything harder to cope with.

THE INABILITY TO DISTINGUISH BETWEEN NIGHT AND DAY

Some people with dementia lose their ability to understand how to tell the time. Many can still actually read the clock and if you ask them will happily say, 'It is 10 o'clock' or whatever is appropriate. However, they do not seem able to understand what this means. Often this does not matter too much and certainly for someone living with a carer who directs and supports them in their daily living, the time is not too important. However, for someone living alone who needs to get to appointments, meet up with others and attend day care, for example, then the ability to read the clock and understand what it means is vital.

Many people with dementia have difficulty in distinguishing between day and night. In the mid-summer months when nights are short and not very dark this can seem logical, but, in fact, whether it is actually dark or not doesn't seem to be significant. Thus families complain that their mother who lives alone is telephoning them at 3 am to complain that no one has visited; a carer's spouse may keep them both awake by insisting on getting out of bed and dressing for the day around midnight. No amount of reasoning, persuasion or pointing out the correct time seems to have any effect and many carers find that the loss of sleep is so debilitating that they feel they can no longer cope with their caring role.

What can I do?

There are some techniques you can try to manage the situation. First, make sure that the person with dementia does not have too many opportunities to sleep during the day. Most people with dementia tend to nod off frequently, particularly as the illness progresses, but you can help to prevent this by planning activities and ensuring that the person gets enough exercise during the day.

Would medication help?

Medication is rarely useful: ordinary sleeping pills do not seem to be effective, but in some cases the hormone **melatonin** has been found to help. This natural product is sometimes used to deal with jet lag and can help to regulate sleep.

Herbal 'sleep remedies' may or may not help. If you live with the person who has dementia you may find that it is better not to get out of bed, even if they do. The fact that you remain in bed may make it clear that it is not time to be up and about and they may return to bed more quickly.

Using full-spectrum daylight bulbs

There is some evidence to show that exposing someone with dementia to full-spectrum daylight for several hours each day will help to 're-set' their biological body clock. Some care homes actually use special full-spectrum daylight bulbs in their residents' lounges to good effect, especially in the dark winter months. You can try this for yourself.

Full-spectrum daylight bulbs are not always readily available in the shops, but can be bought online. You will immediately notice the difference when using these bulbs. The light is white, not yellow, and has been described as like 'putting a window in the room'. Some craft material shops sell full-spectrum daylight lamps that can be angled to provide light on a particular area but it is better to use full-spectrum daylight bulbs in your normal light fittings. Use them for the room where the person with dementia spends most time during the day. Do not use them in the bedroom for obvious reasons.

Safety at night

If you live with someone who gets up at night, you can take steps to ensure their safety by making sure anything harmful is locked away. Switch off kettles and ovens, lock windows and doors and check that there is nothing on the floor that they can trip over. Some carers find that sleeping in a separate room means that they can get some rest even if the person with dementia is up and about.

This wakefulness does not happen to everyone with dementia and many people continue to sleep well at night and keep to a normal body-clock pattern, despite dozing off now and then during the day.

WANDERING AND RESTLESSNESS

Some people with dementia become very restless and begin to pace or to walk around in what appears to be an aimless manner. It is not clear why this habit develops in some people and not in others. In the past this activity was termed 'wandering', but it is now believed that the activity (usually walking around) is not actually aimless and that the person with dementia usually has a purpose in mind – although they may be unable to explain what it is or even to remember it.

Become a detective

If you can, by some clever detective work, find out what is caus-ing the person you care for to engage in frantic activity. You may then be able to forestall the agitation or channel the energy into something more fruitful. For example, when their mind begins to slip back into the past, some people may get anxious that they have forgotten to fetch their children from school or meet their mother after work; they may begin to walk around in an anxious pattern of activity, thinking that they are actually on their way to the school, or doing whatever the anxiety suggests.

Work out the triggers

You won't always be able to discover what is behind the agitated walking, but there are steps you can take to manage it.

If you work out what 'triggers' the behaviour, you can try to avoid this or you can distract the person with dementia when the 'trigger' occurs.

Keeping busy

People with dementia often become bored because the normal activities with which they filled their time are no longer open to them. You can try some of the ideas in chapter 8 to keep boredom at bay (see page 135).

It is a good idea to ensure that the person with dementia has the opportunity for adequate exercise, as agitation may result from a lack of physical activity. Walking, gardening, and some outdoor sports activities, such as bowling or golf, are all good forms of exercise.

If the person you care for continues to walk around in an agitated fashion even after you've tried the tips above, you might consider letting them carry on. Provided they are walking in a safe place (for example, around the garden or in and out of rooms in the house), you can try to ignore the behaviour and not allow it to annoy or worry you – though, easier said than done.

What to do when someone gets lost

Sometimes people with dementia who live alone may set off on a trip to the shops, for example, and then forget where they are going. When this happens they do not usually do what we would consider the 'logical' thing, such as pausing to re-orientate themselves, telephoning a carer, asking someone the way, or stopping until they remember their original aim. Instead, they tend to continue walking and can sometimes walk a considerable distance before they are found by a frantic carer or family, or even the police.

It is generally of no use whatever to try to discover what the original purpose was or to reason with the person who has dementia. Instead, carers should make sure that they know the usual haunts of the person they care for, so that they know where to look first. You can also alert friends and neighbours so that they intercept the person with dementia if they see him/her out alone unexpectedly – or ask them to call you. You could install an alarm that will alert you if an outside door is opened, so that you can stop someone setting off on an unsupervised walk.

Keep a recent photograph of the person with dementia to hand just in case you need to call the police to help look for them.

It is also a good idea to make sure that a person with dementia carries an identification card in their pocket so that if anyone stops to help them they can guide them back home. The Alzheimer's Society has designed a credit-card sized helpcard that states that the person carrying it has a memory problem and might need help. (You can order them from www.alzheimersociety.org or on the phone – see reference section for details.) While most people with dementia do not understand that they can show this card to others if they are lost – and may forget that they even carry the card – police or a helpful passersby may well think to check their pockets for clues and so find it.

It can also be helpful to ensure that the person with dementia carries a mobile phone and that this is always switched on and charged up. People in early-stage dementia may be able to use a mobile if they have used one in the past. Some phones have a single 'emergency' button on the reverse which, when pressed, dials a pre-programmed number or sends a text. But the best thing about a mobile is that it sends out a constant signal that the police can use to 'triangulate' and track down the person with dementia.

There are other electronic devices which can be useful but you need to be careful and thoughtful about the rights of the person you care for – there is a fine balance between best interest and intrusive surveillance. Organisations which can provide electronic solutions are listed in the reference section.

Coping with 'sundowning' – late-afternoon restlessness

The anxiety and restlessness that can overtake people with dementia late in the afternoon is sometimes referred to as 'sundowning' by medical professionals. The person who has dementia begins to become very restless and this may involve walking about, more confusion than normal or bouts of frustrated aggression. Sometimes visual hallucinations or visual disturbances are part of the syndrome. The causes of sundowning are not well understood but the syndrome is extremely stressful for the carer, who is usually tired by late afternoon and looking to wind down and relax. Some research suggests that the agitation may be related to changes to the brain's circadian 'pacemaker' – a cluster of nerve cells that keeps the body on a 24-hour clock. Sundowning is also connected with night wakefulness (discussed above). Sometimes if the problem of night wakefulness is solved restlessness at sundown also disappears.

There is little that doctors or medication can do to help this problem. Exposure to plenty of light during the day may help, especially full-spectrum daylight as detailed above. It can also help to ensure that the person with dementia has plenty of exercise during the day. As twilight comes on and light levels fall, it is good to switch lights on early (ideally with full-spectrum daylight bulbs, as discussed above) and to close the curtains so that the person with dementia is not disturbed by shadows and reflections in the window. Having a meal around twilight may also distract and settle the person with dementia and make them more sleepy.

Carers can try to get some rest or respite earlier in the day so that they are more alert and able to handle this behaviour in the late afternoon/early evening.

Television may make matters worse as early evening news programmes can be very unsettling to someone who is confused. Playing soft gentle music and making the atmosphere as calm as possible is often helpful and some carers have found that if they remain seated, allow the restlessness to 'wash over' them and keep reassuring the person with dementia, the episodes of restlessness get shorter and become less frequent.

COPING WITH INCONTINENCE

The brain governs all our bodily functions and actions and, because the brain in someone with dementia is degenerating progressively, most people who have dementia will become incontinent at some point in the disease. This is very upsetting for those who are caring for them and it can also be upsetting for the person with dementia. Incontinence does not happen at a particular 'stage' in the illness and so it cannot be anticipated.

People with dementia are generally able to manage their own toilet needs at first, although some people may be confused about finding their way to the toilet. This confusion can be helped if you make sure that the location of the toilet is obvious by leaving the door open and the toilet lid up. At night, try leaving a light on in the toilet or bathroom. It's also helpful to make sure that someone with dementia uses the toilet at regular intervals. Frequently you can anticipate a regular bowel movement, thus saving yourself trouble and unpleasantness – it's simply a matter of good timing and observation.

Urinary incontinence usually starts first and it may begin just with the odd 'accident' that carers may put down to being in a strange place, or the person not making it to the toilet in time. But once incidents of incontinence begin they are likely to increase. Sometimes people with dementia are upset and ashamed about their 'accidents' and may try to hide the evidence, tucking wet pants behind radiators or under furniture or making an attempt to mop up or denying that wet patches are anything to do with them. As dementia progresses there is less embarrassment and the person with dementia is likely to allow carers to clean and change them without much sign of awareness of there being any problem.

Incontinence is unpleasant for anyone to deal with and it is often cited as the 'last straw' that pushes families to arrange for residential care in a care or nursing home. However, there are many helpful aids: modern incontinence pads, waterproof pants, bedsheets, bed pads and body wipes are available by mail order and many can be bought at your local pharmacy or supermarket. Special NHS incontinence advisers are supposed to be available in most areas to help with management and the best aids to use, but this service is not always available. Ask your GP or district nursing service whether your area has an incontinence adviser. In some areas they will supply incontinence pads free of charge.

DEALING WITH APPETITE AND WEIGHT LOSS

Variations in appetite are common with dementia because the appetite is controlled by the brain. Some people with dementia develop cravings for certain foods, usually sweet things, and may eat these to excess, even going to the lengths of hiding sweets and biscuits around the house. This can cause problems if the person with dementia also has diabetes and in any case it is not healthy to eat too many sweet and sugary foods. As a carer you may need to be vigilant, but it is no use blaming the person with dementia and getting cross with them if they grab sweets and biscuits, because they are unable to control their craving themselves.

Later in the disease, people with dementia may lose weight and carers can get very concerned about this. The doctor will usually tell you that there is no known reason why weight loss should happen; many people with a serious disease lose weight and it appears that the body is putting all its extra energy into trying to fight the disease, with resulting weight loss. There may also be practical reasons for weight loss. The person with dementia may have a changed sense of taste and no longer find food pleasant to eat. Some people with dementia need constant reminders to eat, even when a meal is placed in front of them. Where people live alone this may mean that they forget to finish a meal or even forget to prepare a meal in the first place.

Some people with dementia forget how to use eating utensils and may eat less because they do not know how to convey the food from plate to mouth. This can be helped by providing 'finger food' or food that is easy to eat, such as sandwiches. As the disease progresses, some people may need to be spoon fed.

If someone with dementia is eating very little, then the carer should try to ensure that everything they do eat has as high a nutritional value as possible. This means using full-fat milk and cheese and eggs and serving high-protein and high-fat food as often as possible. You can fortify food by adding dried milk powder to yogurt and milk drinks, adding cream to soups and sauces, and butter and grated cheese to vegetables. A dietician or nutritional therapist will be able to give specific advice about this – ask your GP for a referral.

(For more on nutrition, see chapter 9, page 153.)

COPING WITH AGGRESSION

Many people associate aggression with dementia but most people with dementia are not habitually aggressive. Any aggression that takes place is usually as a result of frustration at not being able to complete tasks that the person could easily manage before. Some carers find it very difficult to take the right approach to managing a particular person with dementia and this can lead to anger and aggressive behaviour as the person with dementia finds it impossible to express their annoyance in another, more acceptable, way. If the person you are caring for becomes aggressive, it is worth examining your approach to them (see chapter 6, page 107). Ask your dementia support worker, if you have one, or get advice from the community mental health team.

No carer should feel that they have to accept aggressive behaviour, especially if this takes the form of physical violence. It is perfectly reasonable for you to make it clear to the person with dementia that violent or aggressive behaviour is not acceptable. Many people with dementia will calm their behaviour and 'back down' if the carer takes a calm but firm stand.

Certain medication can help to calm someone who is aggressive and carers can always discuss this with the doctor or community psychiatric nurse. In a very few cases hospitalisation is necessary to address this problem. The person with dementia may then need to be 'sectioned' under the Mental Health Act.

COPING WITH LOSS OF INHIBITION

With some forms of dementia people may lose their natural social inhibitions. They may refuse to take their place in a queue, for example, interrupt a conversation, stand too close to someone or do other unacceptable things such as taking their dentures out and showing them to others or exposing their sexual organs.

Not everyone with dementia loses their social inhibitions. Many people retain a sense of what is socially acceptable even after they can no longer remember quite ordinary facts, such as the name of their closest family member. Where loss of inhibition happens it is often the carer who is most upset. Friends and neighbours who know the person with dementia and understand the condition can often cope with strange and otherwise unacceptable behaviour better than close family, who perhaps feel that it is a reflection on them and also are upset by the loss of the person they once knew.

It is perfectly in order to gently remind the person with dementia that a particular behaviour is not socially acceptable and sometimes this is all that is necessary to stop it. At other times, or in a more advanced stage of dementia, you may not be able to prevent socially unacceptable displays.

My husband started to masturbate whenever he was otherwise unoccupied at home. I used to say, 'You can only do that in your own room when you are alone,' and this seemed to stop him each time. If we were out in public it never seemed to happen so I think some social sense did stay with him.

If this behaviour begins after the person you care for moves into a care home, it may be their way of drawing attention to themselves. Unfortunately not all professional carers are trained to understand how to handle this kind of exhibitionism and you may find the managers of the care home complain to you and expect you somehow to deal with this. In these circumstances it is best if you explain how you have handled difficult behaviour at home and point out that boredom or attention-seeking may be playing a part. A good care home with properly trained dementia care workers will be able to manage such behaviour. If the home you have chosen really finds it difficult to deal with, you may like to consider whether you have chosen the best care home.

UNDERSTANDING CLINGING AND DEMANDING BEHAVIOUR

In the earlier stages of dementia, those who are affected may become very demanding of the company of the person closest to them. Although they will probably be unable to reason this out, they are aware that they need their carer and cannot manage without them. The person you care for may begin to feel insecure if you go out of sight or plan to leave them alone even for a short time.

While the person with dementia can still be safely left alone, you can manage this kind of insecurity by being reassuring but firm. State that you have to go out (to do the shopping/to visit the doctor, etc), explain what steps you have taken for their safety and care (there is a sandwich in the fridge, for example, and your mobile phone number is written on the notice board), and reassure them that you WILL return in a specified time. In case of emergency, it is always wise to either let someone know that you will be going out and leaving the person with dementia alone or to carry a card with written details on. Then if something happens – perhaps you have an accident or are delayed – someone can step in to take care of the person with dementia.

In the later stages of the illness it will no longer be safe to leave the person with dementia alone and you may make use of a care-agency worker, a friend or relative or a day centre to allow yourself time for personal matters or essential jobs. Once again, if the person with dementia begins to become upset at being left, you may need to use similar strategies to those mentioned above. You state why you are going out, explain that your 'care substitute' is there to look after them and then calmly leave and return as planned.

It is important not to allow yourself to become virtually 'housebound' because the person you care for becomes upset if you leave them. Make plans and put them into action early in the illness so that the person with dementia becomes used to being left occasionally in the care of others.

Whatever your resolve about caring for a person with dementia at home, in the later stages of dementia you may not be able to cope with difficulties and challenges. While many carers feel guilty about this, the important thing is to work out what you and the person with dementia want from residential care and to ensure the professionals who take over from you are well trained, experienced in dementia care and truly caring.

WHEN IT'S TIME FOR RESIDENTIAL CARE

Most carers set out with the intention of caring for the one they love at home, for as long as it is possible to do so. Most of us, if asked, would say that we would prefer to end our days in our own home surrounded by those things and those people with which we are familiar.

The simple truth is that this is not always possible. The endless demands of caring for someone with dementia may gradually wear the carer down, especially if to a daytime of constant care we add in disturbed nights, the problems caused by incontinence, difficult or aggressive behaviour and the fact that the carer may be elderly and infirm too. Most carers seem to feel a huge sense of guilt about even considering residential care for their loved one and many carry on 'managing' and becoming worn down and depressed and stressed because of this sense of guilt. Support workers understand the effect on carers and can help them to come to terms with feelings of guilt.

Many people have to make a decision about a care home in a crisis, perhaps after a fall or illness, or the death of one half of an elderly couple who was acting as carer. In hindsight, they often wish they'd had longer to choose a home. So if you think the one you care for might need a care home in the future, it's a good idea to start planning sooner rather than later.

Chapter 4

Homes that specialise in caring for those with dementia

These are homes that look after elderly people who are mentally infirm (usually dementia sufferers) and who may or may not be able to manage some of their own personal care but need close supervision – either to stop them getting lost and confused, to prevent them harming themselves, or to help them with every-day living. (Some non-specialist residential care homes and some nursing homes also offer places to a limited number of people with dementia.) People who have dementia without other health complications are not generally considered to need admission to a 'nursing home'.

Nursing homes are a separate category of home. They have a trained nurse on hand at all times. They are able to provide nursing for chronic conditions such as leg ulcers, pressure sores and certain disabilities and conditions (for example, diabetes) where the intervention of a nurse might be required periodically. Not all nursing homes are registered to look after people with dementia who have nursing needs but those that do will be detailed in the local authority lists.

There are particular points to consider where you are looking for a home for someone who has dementia. Many care homes state that they are registered to care for people with dementia and some even state that they are 'specialist' dementia care homes. If a home describes itself as 'specialising in dementia care', then the staff ought to be thoroughly trained in what dementia is, how it affects the brain and in the most caring way to manage the challenges presented by a confused person.

You should not be put off if, when looking round the home, you see people who are particularly affected by dementia. Instead, watch closely to see how these people are cared for: whether members of staff bother to speak to them and pay them attention; whether they are allowed to wander freely if that is what they want to do; and whether there is a variety of activities available that are suitable for them.

How do care home staff manage difficult behaviour?

If staff at the home say that they never experience difficult problems – or if the management tell you that they do not accept people with challenging behaviour – you might want to question how well trained and experienced the staff really are.

A few weeks after my uncle entered the care home I had an urgent call from the managers. They had discovered my uncle in bed with another resident. The lady in question appeared to be perfectly happy and content with the situation. I understood completely that the staff were worried about the lady and what her family would have to say, but I was amazed that, when I asked them how they usually handled such a situation, they said it had never happened before. I found it hard to believe that, in a community where a number of disinhibited people were living together, nothing like this had happened before. What annoyed me most was that I was made to feel somehow to blame – as if my uncle's behaviour was anything to do with me.

Many residential homes claim that their staff are fully trained in managing dementia but there is a wealth of difference between someone who has attended a training course and someone who puts the training into practice and really tries to understand and help those they care for.

I have explained elsewhere in the book that the best way to understand and to help someone with dementia is not to try to force them to conform to the rules of how society thinks they should continue to behave, but rather to understand what and how they are thinking, so that you can work to keep them contented and happy. Well-trained and well-managed staff in a good specialist dementia care home know this.

My wife had a habit of shouting out whenever there was a bit of a bustle around her (like at meal times when people were being moved into the dining room) and the staff at the care home became very annoyed. I discovered that they had asked the doctor to prescribe medication to stop her calling out and this made my wife very sleepy and unresponsive. I wasn't very happy about her being 'drugged up' in this way but the manager of the home told me that the staff were complaining about the shouting and that I either agreed to the drugs or would have to find another home. I began to wonder whether the home was run for the residents or for the convenience of the staff.

When you are looking at care homes ask exactly what kind of training staff have had. It is possible to claim that all staff are 'trained' when all they have done is some on-line training or completed a workbook with multiple choice questions and answers. Ask whether any staff have completed advanced training to become 'dementia champions'. (Note: this is a term used about care-home training and is not to be confused with 'dementia friends champions', which is an initiative to educate people in the wider community about dementia.)

I once tried to discuss personal care problems with workers in a care home. One of the care workers said that she would make a big effort to encourage a resident to have a shower because she [the careworker] always felt better after she had had a shower. The point was that the carer, however well intentioned, was looking at how SHE would feel, NOT at how the person with dementia might feel. Perhaps, instead of feeling clean and refreshed, the resident felt confused, annoyed at being interrupted and violated.

Here are some more examples of managing challenging behaviour:

David is in a long passage with doors on each side. He thinks perhaps he is in a hotel. He starts to open each door looking for his wife. Sometimes there are people in the rooms who shout at him, but he doesn't recognise any room or any person. After a while a woman (a care worker) comes along and stops him saying: 'You mustn't go into other people's rooms.' He wants to ask which is his room but he can't explain properly. The woman walks him a long way to a big room with chairs and makes him sit down. When she has left he gets up and turns back to the passage to find his room.

If David is new to the care home than it would be helpful if someone showed him around – not just once but several times over several days, to help him remember where he is. If he is not new than a care worker could just begin walking with him while discouraging him from opening doors by saying something like: 'Your room is just here, David, at the end of the passage. See, there are all your things.' Or 'Let's go and find your room, David.' David may become less confused when he begins to find his way around or if he understands that the care workers will help him.

Mrs P is wandering happily around the garden of the care home. A care worker comes along and begins to guide her towards the building saying, 'Come along Mrs P, it's time for lunch.'

Mrs P has no conception of the meaning of 'time for lunch'. However, she knows that she is being taken away from her happy wandering and being pressured to go indoors. She struggles and shouts.

Consider how the above situation could be better handled: the care worker begins to walk beside Mrs P, remarking on how nice it is outside. Subtly she guides Mrs P down the path towards the building, perhaps remarking on an attractive flower display. If she pushes open the door and Mrs P smells the lunch cooking she may naturally walk towards the dining room. If she refuses or turns away, the care worker could leave her for a few minutes and try again. Mrs P is happy at that moment and doesn't want that feeling to stop.

What do you and the person you care for want from a care home?

Everyone has different priorities when looking at residential care. Some carers would consider it most important to find the person they care for always washed and dressed and sitting in the lounge when they visit. Others would like to see the person they have always cared for looking happy and wandering around contentedly, even though they may not always be neat and tidy. Still others want to see the person with dementia actively engaged in activities as much as possible. Some carers find it annoying and disturbing if the person they care for is always asleep when they visit. Others are glad of this as it removes the burden of trying to find something to talk about.

It is important to be sure of what you would like to see in your 'ideal' care home, but I hope I have convinced you that the most vital thing is that staff have a good understanding of how to care for someone with dementia and are given the freedom and time by the management to care for your loved one as you would wish them to be cared for.

Chapter 5

Communication

One of the first things often noticed when someone develops dementia is that they become less and less communicative. Spouses will say that they can no longer have a conversation. Family will remark that the person with dementia is quieter and seems less involved in family occasions. Carers notice that the person with dementia no longer initiates a conversation. Sometimes communication difficulties may be spotted long before any formal diagnosis.

My daughter noticed problems with her father's speech and memory 12 years ago. He regularly gave talks and speeches as part of his work and was very frustrated at finding it hard to remember things.

Friends and family often discount such difficulties at first as they seem to be temporary and may be put down to tiredness, depression or 'doing too much'. Sometimes problems may be confused with a sensory condition such as deafness. Perhaps only after the diagnosis of dementia do friends and family begin to look back and recognise symptoms that affected communication and that developed slowly over a period of years.

Communication difficulties are one of the common symptoms of almost all dementias and may involve speech, writing, reading, using a keyboard, understanding the written or spoken word, being able to follow directions or understand symbols (such as road signs) or any combination of these. Not everyone with dementia suffers from problems in all these areas to begin with.

The first thing to remember is that the person with dementia is not refusing to communicate because they do not wish to do so. In nearly every case, people would like to be able to express their thoughts and feelings.

LOSS OF SPEECH

Generally the person with dementia becomes less inclined to speak for one or more of the following reasons:
- they cannot find the right words to say what they want to say
- they cannot follow the conversation so they withdraw from it
- they cannot translate their feelings into words
- they cannot think quickly enough to speak at the right moment
- they think that their difficulties in speaking will result in them being ridiculed
- their speech difficulties make them feel stupid.

Carers, family members and friends can do a great deal to help. There are two very important things to remember and if you only remember these two things you can make a huge difference to communication with the person you care about. They are:
take time
repeat yourself.
Let us examine these two important points in more detail.

TAKE TIME

If you read the section in chapter 1 on the effects of dementia on the brain (see page 3), you will understand that someone with dementia will have a problem with cell connections in their brain.

The nerve cells in the brain are known as neurons. Each neuron has a cell body with a thread-like extension called an axon. Signals pass from neuron to neuron via the axons and have to cross a gap between the axons called the synapse. When the signal reaches the end of the axon it stimulates tiny sacs to release chemicals known as **neurotransmitters** into the synapse. The neurotransmitters cross the synapse and attach to receptors on a nearby cell. In this way the brain sends messages to different parts of the body.

The brain of someone who has dementia will have lost some axons and some of the brain cells will have degenerated, meaning that messages can't always be transmitted via the nerve cells in the normal way. But the human brain is amazingly resourceful and if the obvious route of transmission does not work, it will keep trying until a way is found. This may take some time.

Therefore someone with dementia may take a long time to understand what is being said to them. They may then take an equally long time to formulate a response.

Most conversations happen at a rather fast rate. If you have ever tried to learn a new language and attempted to have a conversation with a native speaker, you may be very aware of this. You may get the gist of what is said but the speaker talks so fast that you cannot keep up. It is possible that the person with dementia has a similar experience. In a situation like this the brain at first tries to keep up with the pace of conversation, but then gives up and seems to 'opt out'. You can also compare this to what happens if a young baby is over-stimulated with games, dangly toys or lots of 'baby talk'. You may notice that the baby 'opts out' and falls asleep when it has had enough – or else starts to yell to let you know.

Slow down

In order to help someone with dementia you should slow down your rate of speech. This can take practice. Often, if we believe someone does not understand what we are saying, our first impulse is to raise our voices. We are all familiar with the cliché that foreigners will understand our language if we only shout loud enough. The other temptation is to speak in a form of 'baby talk'. Neither of these two impulses is helpful when talking to people with dementia – although if they are also hard of hearing, you should of course raise your voice slightly and make sure to face them when you speak.

A steady slowing of your speech will make things easier for the person with dementia. If you listen to experienced care givers – perhaps the spouse of someone who has had dementia for a while – you will notice that they do this automatically. In a mixed group of carers and people with dementia they slip easily from a 'normal' conversational tone with other carers to a steady, slower form of speech when addressing someone with dementia.

If you speak more slowly to someone with dementia, their brain is more likely to process what you have said and they will feel more able to listen and be part of the conversation. In the early days of the illness, people with dementia will sometimes appear irritated if you do this and snap at you, saying something like, 'I'm not stupid you know!' Don't let this put you off. You can acknowledge the comment by saying 'Of course not', but you should continue to keep your rate of speech steady and slower than what we might consider normal. Older people often naturally speak more slowly and for this reason they may find it much easier to converse with someone with dementia.

Use helpful gestures

In addition to slowing your speech, you might like to accompany any questions or directions with helpful gestures (we'll come back to this later in this chapter on page 92). For example, you can pat the chair (not point to it) when you suggest someone sits down. If it is time to leave, you can fetch their coat and hold it up while saying, 'It's time to go now'.

Other helpful gestures include:

- picking up the newspaper when mentioning something you have read in it
- gesturing towards the window if discussing the weather or the garden
- making a drinking gesture when offering a drink
- offering a pen when asking someone to sign something and pointing to the signature line
- touching the garment in question when giving a compliment about clothing.

Remember conversation is a two-way process. The person with dementia has not only to take in and understand what you are saying to them, but to formulate a reply and deliver it coherently. So the second part of the 'take time' tip involves you in doing just that. Having framed your question, suggestion or comment, sit back and give the person with dementia time to respond.

In my work I have been able to observe the way in which someone with dementia responds – often long after one has assumed that the query or comment has passed them by and after the conversation has moved on. It may take several seconds, which can seem like a very long period of silence for the response to be made. As the disease progresses, it can take as much as two minutes to elicit a response. Take the following example:

Care worker: *'Good morning, Mr Jones. How are you today?'*
Carer: *Good morning.*
Care worker: *'It's a lovely day, isn't it?'*
Mr Jones (person with dementia): *'Good morning.'*
Care worker: *'Would you like to take off your coat? Please sit here.'*
(Carer helps Mr Jones to remove coat and guides him to a chair.)
Mr Jones: *'It's nice and sunny today.'*

Notice the gap between the question and the response, and the way in which the person with dementia does actually respond but so slowly that his response and the original question get out of sync.

If you are caring for a family member with dementia, you may soon feel able to deal with conversation in this slower manner, especially when you're at home, so that responses can come in their own good time. However, when out and about even carers may find the silences uncomfortable and start to 'fill' them with small talk, even talking over the person with dementia, so that eventually they either get angry or take the line of least resistance and cease to make the effort to speak.

The best thing then, is to speak slowly and clearly and to allow sufficient time for the person with dementia to formulate and make their response. Sometimes responses may never come. The person with dementia may appear lost in a maze of their own thoughts or they may start to speak and their response drifts away as they find it impossible to find the words they want to use. On some occasions it may help to finish a sentence for someone if you are very sure of what they are trying to say (spouses may be good at this having done it for years, even before dementia set in). Another tactic is to check whether what you've surmised is correct by asking:

'Do you mean ....?'
Or
'Are you talking about.............?'

By slowing your speech and giving ample opportunity for a response, you are giving someone with dementia the attention and dignity they deserve and need – and by your example you may be able to show friends and other family members how to manage a conversation.

REPEAT YOURSELF

The second of these two vital tips is the suggestion that you repeat yourself. You may have noticed children doing this all the time.

'Mum, can I have some sweets? Can I have some sweets? I want some sweets. Mum. Mum. Can I have some sweets?'

They seem to know instinctively that a response (even if a pretty short-tempered one) will eventually come with this tactic.

One of the main symptoms of any form of dementia is the loss of short-term memory. This generally refers to very short-term memory so that someone with dementia may ask you the same question several times in succession even though you have just supplied an answer.

Person with dementia: *'Are we going out today?'*
Carer: *'Yes. We're going round to Fred's house after breakfast.'*
Person with dementia: *'OK.'*
(Carer continues to eat breakfast.)
Person with dementia: *'Are we going out today?'*
Carer: *'I have just told you we are going to Fred's house after breakfast.'*
Person with dementia: *'Where?'*
Carer: *'To Fred's house – after breakfast.'*
Person with dementia: *'OK.'* (Eats a few mouthfuls of food.) *'Are we going out today?'*
Carer (exploding with impatience): *'I've told you twice that we are going to Fred's. Why don't you listen?'*
Person with dementia: *'Going to Fred's? Today?'*

The person with dementia is truly not trying to make life difficult or deliberately annoying you. They have forgotten that they have asked the question and forgotten the answer. But the impulse to ask the question is still there. They are sure that they want to know something.

So the second tip is: repeat yourself.

Generally we try to avoid repeating ourselves too often, although it is actually quite a natural thing to do. Teachers are advised to repeat themselves at least three times – 'Tell them what you are going to say; say it; tell them what you said' – on the premise that it needs at least three repetitions for the average person to remember something. But someone who has dementia has great difficulty in remembering. So how many times should you repeat things for them? Is there a magic number? Of course not.

Many health professionals are taught to repeat their instructions because it is known that this repetition helps any patient to follow an instruction. For example, an optometrist may tell you to look straight ahead when he or she is examining your eyes. You may notice that the optometrist repeats this command as he or she continues the examination. This is because of the natural human trait to 'wander' from the instruction. Although you begin by looking straight ahead and although you fully intend to keep looking straight ahead until told otherwise, your brain has other ideas and it quickly loses the concentration needed to keep looking straight ahead and starts to flick around looking in every direction. By repeating the command to 'look straight ahead' at intervals, the optometrist brings the brain's attention back and keeps you looking where required. Similarly the dentist's command to 'open a bit wider, please' brings your attention back when your jaw has started to slacken.

Keep up a running commentary

We know how much harder it is for someone with dementia to command their own attention span; they will be more inclined to forget what has been said and to need reminding. We may avoid giving repeated reminders because we know that they would be very annoying if given constantly to us. However, this is not the case for someone with dementia. They have a shorter attention span so they may not take in all that is said in the first place. Secondly, because they have a faulty short-term memory, they are likely to forget what has been said very quickly. Constant reminders are not annoying to someone with dementia. On the contrary they are most helpful – always provided they are given without impatience and in the right tone.

> *'We are going out shopping now. Let's get our coats.'*
> *'Here is your coat. We are going out shopping.'*
> *'Are you ready? We are going shopping now.'*
> *'Hope we get to the shops before it rains.'*
> *'Here we are. Let's get our shopping.'*

At first this level of repetition seems artificial and may even annoy you, the carer. However, with continual practice it can become almost automatic and you will find yourself able to keep up this kind of running commentary very well. The person you are caring for will not find your repetition annoying because they have forgotten each time you say something that you have said it.

Another tactic is to find different ways of saying the same thing.

> *'John is coming to lunch today.'*
> *'Look out for John – he's coming to lunch.'*
> *'I have to start making lunch because John is coming today.'*

'I am making shepherd's pie for lunch because John is coming.'
'Can you help lay the table for lunch? John will be here soon.'
'Are you looking forward to seeing John when he comes to lunch today?'

Actions speak louder than words

As dementia progresses, it is helpful to use actions as well as words and to make use of as many senses as possible. For example, use gestures much more than you might normally. Pull out the chair in which you want someone to sit, pat the table on which you want them to place something, hold up the book or newspaper you are referring to, pick up the coat you want them to put on, and so forth. People with dementia may understand much better if you 'show as well as tell'. As an example, if you want someone with advanced dementia to understand that it is time for bed you might hold up their pyjamas or nightdress and say 'Time for bed now.'

People with dementia often lose the impulse to wash and dress themselves quite early in the illness. This is probably because their 'executive function' is damaged (see chapter 1 on the brain in dementia) or it may be because they have lost the ability to follow a sequence when carrying out an action. It can be very helpful to start the action off by, for example, undoing buttons on a shirt or jacket to indicate that it is time to undress. Or you might walk the person with dementia into the bathroom and switch on the shower to 'trigger' the actions needed to take a shower. In doing this it is important not to pull or push someone around without ceremony. No one wants to be forcibly made to take action. The best thing is to take someone gently by the arm and walk them towards the shower, for example, or to begin unfastening clothes while keeping up a simple conversation (preferably one that doesn't require them to concentrate on finding answers).

Sometimes people with dementia lose their orientation quite early on in the disease. They may stand around looking confused, walk in the wrong direction or not seem to understand when you direct them to a chair or when you give instructions about where to go. The kindest thing is simply to take their arm and show them where to go in a gentle and unobtrusive manner. Instructions like 'turn left' or 'go across the road' or 'follow that path' don't seem to help at all, and maps and plans seem to lose their meaning. A set of directions is unlikely to be understood in full or to be followed properly.

Leaving notes

Written notes can help for a limited time. Some carers find that putting a note in a prominent place helps the person they are caring for if they have to be left alone. For example:

'Jill has gone to the shops and will be back before lunch.'

Notes like this may be helpful if the person you are caring for can safely be left alone but gets worried if you are away too long. However, as the disease progresses such written instructions are less helpful. People with dementia can often retain the ability to read (and read aloud) the written word for a long time but they seem to lose the ability to understand what they are reading or to interpret it in a meaningful way. Similarly, carers find that written instructions for using an appliance like the washing machine, for example, may be of use only for a limited time.

Learn to measure time in different ways

Similarly, you may find that although the person you care for may still be able to read the time on a clock, they do not understand its meaning. To convey when something is going to happen it is more helpful to associate it with another event. For example, in a day centre the carers are unlikely to say 'The bus will be here to collect you at 4 o'clock,' but rather 'The bus will be along after tea.' You can use a similar tactic and say things like:

'We will be going to bed after supper.'
'We will be going round to see Susan after we have been to the library.'

Keep a day book

If someone with dementia is living alone it can help if you begin to get them used to using a big (preferably brightly coloured) book in which to write things down. Start off this system as soon as you can after the illness has been diagnosed, so that you both get into the habit of using the book and keeping it in the same place (such as on the hall table). Write down everything. Here are some examples:

Change sheets on Wednesday
Chiropodist will come on Tuesday afternoon
Dentist appointment Friday
Leave post out for Sally to check
Sandwiches for lunch are in the fridge.

If you can get the person you care for to get used to this system in the early stages of the disease it can work for a long time, until eventually they can no longer understand written instructions. An aid as simple as this book can enable someone to continue to live alone in their home for longer than would otherwise be the case.

Be sure to write important telephone numbers in the front of the book, but keep the list short. If you, the carer, always make health appointments for the person with dementia, don't confuse them with a long list that includes the dentist, optician, chiropodist and so on. Include your own number and that of any other family member or neighbour who can help if called upon at short notice.

Make use of pictures and photos

Pictures may work for longer than words. Try sticking pictures of people next to their speed-dial number on the phone, for example. Putting pictures of cups, plates, etc, on kitchen cupboards can sometimes help someone with dementia who gets confused by all the closed cupboards in the kitchen. Some carers put a picture of a toilet bowl on the bathroom door to help with orientation.

Top tips for successful communication

If possible, always **face the person you are talking to** and **get down (or up) to their level. Use names** to attract attention. For example, instead of saying:

'Would you like a cup of tea, John?'
Say:
'John [this gets his attention], *would you like a cup of tea?'*

If you do not see the person with dementia every day, get into the habit of identifying yourself each time you meet.

'Hello John, I'm Elizabeth.'

Identifying yourself like this does no harm and will give a gentle reminder without drawing attention to a memory problem.

If you are talking about someone else, use their name often – rather than referring to them as 'he' or 'she'.

For example, say: *'Give the apples to Sarah.'*
Rather than: *'Give her the apples.'*

Be thoughtful when asking questions

I would like to reiterate the suggestion given in an other chapters that you avoid too many questions and particularly avoid complex questions. When anyone asks us a question we have to process a lot of information. We have to realise that a question is being asked – if we do not have dementia this is usually obvious. We have to understand the question and if we don't, we may ask for clarification by saying something like, 'What do you mean?' or, 'Do you mean such and such?' Then we have to decide what we want to say in reply – because, of course, a straight question doesn't always warrant a straight answer. Finally, we have to frame our answer in words and deliver it verbally.

For the person with dementia all these stages are difficult. When someone has dementia their thought processes are slower. This does not mean that they are stupid or incapable of thought; it means that the process takes longer. It takes longer in the first place to realise that they are being addressed. Usually we realise we are being spoken to because the person addressing us looks directly at us, possibly uses our name and probably asks the question as a result of a previous interaction.

It takes longer for a person with dementia to realise that a question has been asked. Conversation takes quite a lot of concentration. Distractions in the form of other people around, background noise and so on, do not help.

Processing the question takes longer for a brain in which the neurons that convey signals to one another are wasting away or firing in a random pattern.

Deciding on an answer takes longer for the same reason. In addition, many people with dementia have difficulty in framing words, in putting words together to make coherent sentences and in saying what they actually mean.

The end result is that answering questions is very stressful for someone with dementia.

Chapter 5

Making decisions

This does not mean that we should never ask questions. It is good for someone with dementia to have some control over their surroundings and to make choices. The Mental Capacity Act states that a person's mental capacity must be judged according to the decision that needs to be made. It is no longer acceptable for a doctor to make a blanket statement that a person 'does not have capacity'. Someone may not have the mental capacity to decide whether they should move into a care home but they are still perfectly capable of deciding whether they'd like tea or coffee.

However, questions should be kept simple, should be framed clearly and should be answerable within the abilities of the person with dementia (see page 80).

Interpreting cries for help

In the later stages of dementia some people may have extreme difficulty in framing sentences. This may mean that their communication takes the form of expletives (such as swear words) or of simple staccato phrases like 'no' or 'help me' or 'it's awful'. These phrases are not meaningless. When someone with dementia speaks they are attempting to communicate as best they can. It helps to remember that in these late stages the structured, logical form of thinking is almost completely lost but that the emotional reactive thinking is still very much in evidence.

When someone has dementia their ability to think logically and to follow a reasoned argument is gradually lost. However, the ability to feel emotions is not lost and so reactions tend to be emotional ('I am happy'; 'I am cross') rather than logical ('I am feeling fed up because I did not sleep well and I have to go to the dentist today'). The Alzheimer's Society has a very good 'bookshelf model' which demonstrates this change in thinking on the website www.alzheimers.org.uk

What does this mean in practice?

89

When someone with dementia says 'no', they probably mean that they do not want to be put to the effort of engaging with you. 'No' is a very powerful word – which may be why babies seem to learn it early in their development. In general, if someone – including someone with dementia – says 'no', the person attempting to interact with them will stop trying.

Let us consider the case of someone with dementia living in a care home and who says 'no' persistently when the care worker is asking them if they want breakfast.

'Bill, do you want your breakfast now?'

'No.' (I don't know what she is asking. I don't understand; but when I say no she leaves me alone.)

What would happen if the care worker asks the same question while offering Bill a plate of bacon and eggs? Perhaps he would still say 'no' because that is all he is able to say, but he might grab the plate, or sit at the table because the 'food is ready' message is getting through.

What might happen if the care worker simply put the food on the table and said, 'Here is your breakfast, Bill,' while pulling out his chair and indicating that he should sit?

What might happen if the care worker arranged to have Bill sitting at the table and spread his napkin over his knees and got his knife and fork ready and only then put the food on the table, saying, 'Here is your breakfast, Bill'?

'Help me' or just 'Help!' is another common phrase that people with dementia seem to use when they are in the advanced stage of dementia. In some care homes the staff try their hardest to find out what the problem is by asking the person calling out what they want or need. If they get no response or cannot discover what they need, staff will begin to simply ignore the shouts for help. In one care home one person with dementia called out so loudly and so often that the neighbours in houses next door regularly asked the manager to 'Please help that poor lady.'

As with the constant response of 'no', the cry for help is expressing a need. It is often impossible to discover what's wrong by attempting to ask the person with dementia. The truth is they can no longer express themselves enough to say what they want. If they could, they would make themselves clear – even if not in exact words. Their vocabulary is now limited to expletives and simple phrases. Like the word 'no', the words 'help me' are a very simple and basic expression.

Care staff may have to use all their powers of deduction to establish what's wrong – but they should be under no illusion that the crying out is not expressing a need. First it helps to establish when the crying for help happens. If you ask staff they will often claim it happens 'all the time' or 'at random', but this is seldom the case. If staff note down every time the shouting out occurs, a pattern will probably establish itself. Perhaps the person with dementia calls for help when they see the bustle of meal times as everyone is moved into the dining room. Perhaps the crying out occurs when they are being bathed or washed – maybe the person with dementia feels they are being violated or that their space is being invaded.

The crying out may occur particularly at busy times or especially when everything is quiet – have they been forgotten? It may happen only when there are visitors around or when the television is on – is it too noisy? Or if they are outside in the garden – what is this place? Crying for help may happen at different times of day and on different occasions, but analysis often establishes what these times and occasions are.

Once the pattern of crying out has been established it may be good to have a 'team think' about why it is happening. Often the family and friends know the history of the person with dementia and they may come up with the answer as they describe what the person they used to know was like.

'Mum always hated too much noise.'
'She couldn't bear a mess around her.'

'Dad was a keen gardener. Maybe he wants to do some weeding.'
'My aunt never liked cold food.'
'He likes a bath. I don't think he ever had a shower in his life.'

It may take several attempts but frequently the trigger that causes the crying out can be identified. It may not always be possible to prevent someone crying out for help, but at least this kind of analysis can establish how to help when it happens.

Dealing with swearing

Swearing and cursing, although socially unacceptable, are simply another way of trying to communicate for someone with advanced dementia. Usually it will indicate disapproval and annoyance, but it may simply be the only words that can be expressed in the later stages. People who have been in certain occupations (the armed forces is one example) may have been used to hearing swear words used routinely at work until such words became the norm in that situation. When you take into account that people with dementia have lost their most recent memories, together with many social inhibitions, it is not surprising that swear words are used. We should also remember that swear words are emotional words and so when thinking and expression have become purely emotional in nature due to the progression of dementia, these are the words that are used. Although carers may express shock at hearing such words, this will not stop the person with dementia swearing. Again, what is needed is to work out what emotion (usually anger or annoyance) is being expressed and the reason for this.

Interpreting gestures and facial expressions

When verbal expression is lost or almost lost, carers need to become more aware of body movements, facial expressions and other signs that express communication. If someone pushes aside a proffered cup of tea it may be because they do not want a drink; untrained staff will use this as an excuse to simply remove the cup – consequently the person with dementia doesn't get enough to drink. However, the person with dementia may not be refusing the drink. They may prefer a different drink. Alternatively, they may not understand what they are being offered. It may take some time for them to recall what to do with a cup of liquid. It can help for the care worker to sit down beside them and perhaps place their hands around the cup. It may be helpful if the person pushing aside the cup can sit somewhere where they can see others using cups to drink from, so that they are reminded of what the cup is for. It can help for a care worker to gently remind them several times to 'drink your tea'. It may simply be that the tea is too hot to drink. Several alternatives may have to be tried before the gesture of pushing aside the cup is recognised for what it is.

Emotional responses

Even in advanced dementia, people still feel emotion. Indeed, as dementia advances, the logical factual abilities give way to a more emotional way of thinking. The person with dementia may not be able to explain that a care worker seems like an authority figure and reminds them of a teacher they hated and feared, but this fear will be the uppermost emotion in their mind when that particular care worker approaches them. Often care workers take it as a personal insult if a person with dementia seems not to like them. This means that they have had insufficient training in the facts about dementia. Someone with dementia thinks emotionally and cannot help themselves. A trained care worker should think rationally and be able to understand that these emotional reactions are not within the control of the person with dementia. She or he should allow another worker to take over in such situations without resentment and without feeling upset.

Conversely, someone with dementia may especially enjoy the help provided by a particular care worker because in their emotional thought processes they see them as comforting and nurturing – like a mother figure, for example. This explains why someone with dementia may, for example, mistakenly call their carer 'Mum' or 'Nurse' when they are helping them to get dressed in the morning – the person with dementia is responding to their emotions, which tell them that mothers – and nurses – are caring people.

Another example of an emotional response would be when someone with dementia needs help to use the toilet, but they are not be able to understand this and their emotions may tell them that having their skirts lifted up or their trousers pulled down by others is not an acceptable thing to happen. They may become indignant and start to struggle and shout.

Within the family these late stages of dementia may be even more difficult. As emotional thinking takes over, long unacknowledged feelings of resentment or dislike may surface – feelings that parents or children disguised or repressed previously in the interests of good care and harmony. A mother who resented her daughter but suppressed this feeling because she felt it incompatible with being a good parent, may now become angry and begin to say unpleasant things to her daughter. A previously loving husband may start to say upsetting and hurtful things to his wife.

It is very trying for someone who has been caring for a long time and has perhaps put their own life 'on hold' for the good of the person with dementia, only to find expressions of resentment and apparent hatred coming their way instead of gratitude for the care they give. It can be impossible for the carer to ignore the things that are said and even if they are able to tell themselves that the person with dementia is unaware of the hurt they are causing, carers are still very likely to be upset and to need extra support from friends and family. The difficulty is that people with dementia may be pleasant and sociable with outsiders (friends and neighbours), so that they find it difficult to believe the resentful behaviour and the unpleasant things that are said in private. Carers should do their best to get as much respite as they can and should also be assured that support workers from organisations such as the Alzheimer's Society and Carers' Support really do understand the situation and can provide a listening ear.

It is reported that two thirds of communication is non-verbal[1] and this becomes more apparent as dementia progresses. Carers can become proficient at understanding what the person they care for wants to communicate, even after speech becomes almost non-existent. As the disease progresses non-verbal methods of communication and emotional thinking become more important than intellectual speech and rational thought processes. Understanding this progression will help both carers and people with dementia to live meaningful lives together.

1. Hogan K, Stubbs R (2003). *Can't get Through - 8 Barriers to Communication.* Grenta, LA: Pelican Publishing Company.

Chapter 6

Making changes to your own behaviour

When to do this, how to do this and how to decide when it is necessary

As I have described in chapter 1 and chapter 5, people with dementia have a problem with the cognitive processes of their brain, which means that they take longer to process information and sensory input. After a time they may become unable to process any new information or to learn new things. This makes life very stressful for them – and of course for you, the carer.

This means that the normal ways of communicating, of reasoning, of explaining and presenting a meaningful argument, no longer work when dealing with someone who has dementia.

Living and associating with another person require a constant active compromise. We adjust our habits, our actions and our conversation in the interest of 'rubbing along together', even though we may not realise we are doing this. Over many years these actions and adjustments become habitual, but they still remain. In any social situation everyone is involved in this constant compromise. Of course we know that most relationships are unequal and one member of the relationship may make more adjustments than the other, but living with or simply associating with someone involves a constant daily compromise between pleasing ourselves and pleasing someone else.

People who have dementia gradually lose their ability to

see another person's point of view: they lose their ability to empathise, to understand the everyday compromises that kept the partnership going. The carer is left making all the compromises and possibly without even the satisfaction of a shared sense of humour, as one example, that they formerly enjoyed – and certainly without the sense of support they might have had in the past from their partner.

Many carers take a long time to accept that the past methods of working through a problem or a dilemma, or of resolving a difference of opinion, no longer work. Some never realise this and their relationship with the person who has dementia is doomed to be full of strife and argument. The carer will be angry and frustrated and feel guilty. The person with dementia will be angry and frustrated and feel misunderstood. In an effort to make their point, the person with dementia may resort to anger, abuse and even violence. Social services or even the police may need to intervene, and the person with dementia may be sectioned under the Mental Health Act – with all the associated distress, unnecessary medical intervention and guilty remorse.

It is vital that you, the carer, accept that, soon after the diagnosis of dementia, you are going to have to change your behaviour – in particular your methods of communication – to accommodate the reduced level of understanding and reasoning that the person with dementia now has.

This is not an easy thing to do. Oddly enough, professional paid carers can achieve this more easily (although they do not all manage to do so) because their relationship with the person with dementia is not personal. However, when the carer and the person with dementia have known each other well and for a long time they know exactly how to irritate each other, how to provoke and annoy. It takes a strong and understanding carer to break out of this pattern of behaviour and to rise above it, calmly and patiently – to create, as far as possible, a stress-free environment.

I am going to give you some tips that will help you do this. They are simple suggestions but they will work IF you can adapt and use them.

Relationships without dementia involve give and take, even if they are never entirely equal. With dementia the ability to 'give' goes and the sufferer cannot do anything about this – the carer does all the giving and the person with dementia does all the taking. There are, however, ways of making this unavoidable situation less stressful for both carer and cared-for.

1. Accept that YOU need to change YOUR behaviour

This is probably the hardest thing to do. The person who has dementia is no longer able to reason or plan their reactions. They have an illness that makes this impossible. (You can re-read the section on how dementia affects the brain to understand why this is so.)

You must accept this. To make adaptations in behaviour it is necessary to be able to reason, to think things out and to plan ahead. If you find yourself continually thinking that the person with dementia is 'doing it deliberately' or 'trying to wind me up', you may never manage a peaceful co-existence and your future with the person who has dementia is bound to be difficult.

'Hold on!' I can hear you saying already, 'Why is it all down to me? My husband/wife/ mother/father must make some effort surely? Life is about compromise. It will be impossible for me to spend my whole time adapting my behaviour.'

Well, the truth is that of course the person with dementia will also have to compromise, but the way in which this will work will be explained later in this chapter (see 'Do not let yourself be bullied or intimidated' (page 107)). For now, accept that YOU must change your behaviour – you will find that the rewards in terms of reduced stress are worth it.

2 . Do not ask complex questions

There are some people who believe that you should refrain from asking the person with dementia any questions at all, but this extreme action is not necessary.

As I explained in chapter 5, when someone asks us a question we have to process a lot. We have to realise that a question is being asked. If we do not have dementia this is usually obvious. We have to understand the question. If we do not have dementia and we do not quite understand we may clarify by saying something like, 'What do you mean?' or, 'Do you mean such and such?' We have to decide what we want to answer because of course a straight question doesn't always warrant a straight answer. Finally, we have to frame our answer in words and deliver it verbally.

For the person with dementia all these stages are difficult. When someone has dementia their thought processes are slowed. This does not mean that they are stupid or incapable of thought. It means that the process takes longer. All this means that *questions are very stressful for someone with dementia*.

This does not mean that we should never ask questions. It is good for someone with dementia to have some control and to make choices. Keep questions simple, frame them clearly and make sure the answer is within the capabilities of the person with dementia.

Look at the following contrasting examples.

> *'What would you like? We have tea, coffee or perhaps you would prefer a cold drink?'*

A simpler, better way to frame the question would be:

> *'Would you like a drink?'*

Wait for the answer – a simple yes or no; if yes, follow up with:

Chapter 6

'Would you like tea or coffee?'

Another example:

'Shall we go for a walk or would you rather go to the shops?'

Better alternative:

'Let's go for a walk?' (Note here that although you have turned the question into a proposal, the person you are talking to still has the option to say 'no'.)

3 . Reduce the choices on offer

This goes hand in hand with simplifying how you ask questions. Complex choices make someone with dementia confused and panicky. They may respond by refusing to make a choice at all, by making a random choice that they regret or by getting angry.

Carers often tell me the person they are looking after takes too long to do something. For example:

'I told him to go and change his shirt and 20 minutes later he still hadn't done it.'
'My wife spends a long time every morning going through her wardrobe pulling out clothes and then replacing them aimlessly.'
'My mother can't even make a cup of tea. She opens the food cupboard and just stares at it helplessly.'

All these difficulties are the result of too much choice. You can make life simpler by handing out the clean shirt to be worn, by taking two garments from the wardrobe and offering a simple choice between them, by clearing the cupboard of everything except the tea-making ingredients. Remember at no time will you be preventing the person with dementia from making a

101

choice. Even though you are reducing their options, they can still reject the shirt you give them, refuse the two dresses you show them, decide not to make tea.

By reducing the number and complexity of choices to be made you are actually empowering the person with dementia: you are giving them the satisfaction of making a choice without the stress associated with too many alternatives.

4 . Do not contradict

No one likes being contradicted but we usually accept it – perhaps because whoever is correcting us is right, or because we don't want to cause an argument.

When someone has dementia they may tell an anecdote or story in a muddled or confused way or they may be confused in their recall and relate something that is actually wrong. If you contradict them, they are likely to become even more confused, and to have their confidence reduced. They may become angry because they feel you are belittling them. You may think it is important to 'put them right', but in actual fact it seldom matters. If the listeners know that the person telling the story has dementia they will be able to discount details that do not add up. If they do not realise that the person has dementia, then you can quietly take them aside and indicate the truth without drawing undue attention to the fact.

This is another instance where you as the carer can get the impression that the feelings of the person with dementia are being given consideration above yours. But once again, you should accept that this is a necessary compromise to reduce stress all round.

It can be worth comparing the actions taken to reduce stress for someone with dementia to the actions you would happily take if the person you are caring for had another serious illness – for example, diabetes. If you were caring for someone with diabetes, you would keep an eye on their medication and ensure that they did not eat too many of the wrong kinds of food, because all these actions are important in caring for a diabetic. Dementia of any kind is a serious illness and reducing stress is an important feature of the treatment. You would not ignore relevant treatment if you were caring for someone with diabetes just because it inconvenienced you, so why neglect to support someone who has dementia in order simply to save your 'feelings'?

Mr M felt very aggrieved because his wife kept suggesting that her father had carried out various DIY jobs around the house, when in actual fact he had done so. He told me that they had endless arguments because he tried to explain to her that she was wrong (her father had died many years before). I suggested that what she said was not really very important, but he replied: 'It is to me. I spent hours on those repairs.' After some discussion he agreed to try not to get annoyed and to simply say, 'Did he?' the next time his wife said 'My father repaired that...' A few weeks later he reported that he had been able to ignore his hurt feelings and that his evenings were now much more pleasant because he did not spend time trying to make his wife understand the facts. He was later able to rationalise that he had always been slightly jealous of his wife's affection for her father and that this had coloured his attitude to something that he agreed was really of little importance.

5. Do not criticise

As dementia progresses the person you are caring for will become less able to carry out everyday activities. It is not a matter of 'not trying'. We would all prefer to be independent and no one really chooses to be bathed, dressed or led around by another person, however kindly this is done. Indeed, the person with dementia may insist that they can carry out some activities long after it is clear that they can no longer do so and they may become angry when help is offered.

It follows then that criticising their lack of ability is unhelpful. It is better to be matter-of-fact and to give help in an unobtrusive way than to draw attention to their lack of ability.

Never discuss this decline in abilities with someone else while the person with dementia is within earshot. Although often the person with dementia may give the appearance of not taking in what you are saying to someone else, they will often be aware from your body language and from the tone of your voice that you are speaking about them and perhaps denigrating their abilities.

6. Decide what is really important

When you are caring for someone with dementia, life can seem like a constant battle. You may need to insist that they bathe, change their clothes, eat properly and behave appropriately. You may need to stop them from doing something dangerous, to help them to manage their finances and to take over everyday chores that were previously their responsibility. Needing to do some or all of these things can be really tiring and if, in addition, you have to manage awkward behaviour (a refusal to wash, for example) or the person with dementia insisting that they can manage alone when you know they cannot, you may often feel stressed and exhausted. Even if the person you are caring for is compliant and accepting of help, the constant supervision and attention required can exhaust you.

The first thing to do is to decide what is essential, what is important, and what does not really matter. You may be surprised to discover when you analyse things that there are fewer essentials than you previously thought.

Take the example of hygiene. Most of us have a bath or shower on most days because we find it pleasant to do so – we feel fresher

– and because we have been educated to believe that a daily bath or shower is essential. We might like a shower to wake us up in the morning or a warm bath to prepare for bed at night. In fact, a daily bath or shower is not necessary for cleanliness. Think about this. How do we know that someone is dirty? Either we can see dirt on their skin or clothes or we detect an unpleasant odour which indicates they have not washed for a while.

If the person you care for is becoming reluctant to have a daily bath or shower, you may be keen to carry on encouraging them to do so, but provided the person you care for is not incontinent (when a daily shower or bath will be more important), then a simple wash may be perfectly adequate.

Many of us like to wash our hair on a daily basis and become very upset if the person we are caring for refuses to wash their hair or even to have it washed. Again, we should consider how often a hair wash is really necessary.

The best way to illustrate how you can decide what is essential, what is important and what does not really matter is to examine some case studies.

Case study: Margaret

Margaret is an 82-year-old woman with dementia. She lives alone and her main carer is her daughter Sally, who is the youngest daughter in the family and who lives nearby. Sally also looks after her husband, who is disabled, and her teenage children. Sally is worried about Margaret's diet because Margaret is no longer able to cook and Sally believes that she does not eat regularly.

Sally believes that a proper diet which incorporates three meals a day and plenty of fruit and vegetables is **essential**. In order to work out whether this is so, we need to look at the facts. We check that Margaret is not losing weight. (Although Margaret resists being weighed, Sally confirms that Margaret's usual clothes still fit her: they are no looser or tighter than previously –

so she hasn't gained any weight either.) Apart from the dementia, Margaret is normally healthy and does not have an excessive number of colds or infections.

We can conclude therefore that Margaret's diet is not so bad that she is losing weight or becoming ill. However, Sally would like to ensure that Margaret stays well so we conclude that paying attention to Margaret's diet is **important**.

Case study: Bill

Bill has dementia. He lives with his wife, Audrey, who gets upset when Bill often does not seem to recognise her and calls her by the name of their eldest daughter. Audrey feels that Bill sometimes does this to annoy her because on other occasions he knows she is his wife. Audrey also feels very hurt by the fact that after a marriage of more than 50 years she is 'not recognised' and she thinks it is **important** that Bill calls her by her correct name.

Let's look at the facts again. Bill's dementia means that his brain is 'misfiring' in a random manner. He has difficulty remembering names. However, he does not use a random name when addressing Audrey. He either calls her by her name or (on occasion) uses the name of their eldest daughter. This indicates that Bill realises that Audrey is a close member of his family. He does recognise Audrey, he just calls her by the wrong name. He is not doing this to annoy her. He recognises that she is someone who is important to him. When Audrey understands this she realises that the error is not important. **It does not really matter**.

Case study: Frances

Frances has dementia and lives with her husband. She no longer recognises the time or the difference between day and night. Often in the night Frances will wake up, get out of bed and roam about the house. On occasion she has opened the front door and wandered

outside. Usually her husband wakes up before this happens and manages to get her back to bed. If Frances
were to go out she might get lost or walk out into traffic.
Her husband needs to be aware of when she gets
out of bed and especially if she opens the door and
attempts to go outside. **This is essential**.

These case studies are typical of the kind of problems that carers
face. If you are able to step back and view the things that are worrying
you in the same manner, you may conclude that many of the things
you considered essential or important do not really matter. Letting
go of unimportant things will help to make you less stressed and will
ease your relationship with the person with dementia.

7. Do not let yourself be bullied or intimidated

Perhaps this tip is a surprise to you! Up until now it seems that
all the suggestions have been aimed at you, the carer, adapting
to the person with dementia. This is rightly so. The person who
has dementia cannot reason and cannot understand the need to
adapt in order to make life run smoothly. This is not their fault.
They have an illness which affects the part of the brain which
generally allows them to adapt their behaviour in this way.

However, I want to emphasise two things. As a carer, you have
the right to a stress-free and quiet life – but at the same time you
must act in a way that is in the best interests of the person with
dementia.

Acting in someone's best interests does NOT mean allowing
them to do what they like, especially if this is dangerous or
likely to upset others. Think about how you would manage a
child's behaviour. Children are not experienced enough in life
to understand what is best for them. For example, a child may
well protest at having to go to bed even though they are tired
and need to get plenty of sleep to cope with school the next day.

I am NOT suggesting that an adult with dementia is like a

child, but the part of their brain that allows them to think ahead and work out how their actions may affect themselves or others is damaged. As a carer you need to think about what is in their best interests. If we saw someone with dementia about to step out into a busy road without checking the traffic (something which seldom happens, incidentally), we would intervene straight away and stop them. This is a simple example of acting in the best interests of the person with dementia – although possibly they might get angry with us for interfering and not be glad that we had saved them from danger.

Although I have suggested that you do not criticise or contradict the person with dementia, this does not mean that you should allow them to ride roughshod over another person's feelings or to ignore their needs. We have already seen that the person with dementia can often not be reasoned with and that persuasion frequently results in their becoming more stubborn. So, you may be wondering, how do you manage difficult behaviour?

You manage by making it clear that you will not put up with anti-social behaviour. In order to do this you must 'stand back' from any emotional involvement with the person who has dementia, as far as this particular behaviour is concerned. You must not get angry or embarrassed or break down in tears. None of these things will be effective. You must state clearly and calmly that a particular behaviour will not be tolerated. For example:

'You cannot drive the car. Your licence has been revoked and it is against the law.'
'Hitting people is not allowed.'
'You must pay for sweets [in the shop] before you eat them.'
'Do not swear at me.'
'You must not shout at the neighbours.'

Think carefully about which behaviours you take a stand against. It is important that the person with dementia does not hit other people – this could lead to a complaint and even to police involvement. It is not really important if they refuse to wear gloves when it is cold. It is important that the person with dementia does not abuse or attack you; it is not really important if they do not wish to take a daily bath or shower. It is important that the person with dementia does not step out into the road without looking; it is not important if they refuse to eat the meal you have just cooked (unless they are diabetic and have just taken their insulin, of course).

Sometimes the person with dementia has always been the dominant person in a relationship – that's a normal part of life. This is quite acceptable whilst all parties in the relationship are amenable to this and understand one another, but there is a point beyond which dominance becomes bullying and it is unacceptable to allow yourself or other family members to be bullied by someone who is no longer capable of understanding their own best interests or yours.

Families often find it very difficult to take a stand and they tiptoe around the person with dementia, allowing them to rule the roost because they are afraid to do otherwise. Naturally no one wants to cause an unpleasant scene or provoke violence, but there is a time when you need to stand back and decide whether such behaviour is in anyone's best interests.

Mum had become very difficult, refusing to leave the house, or to allow Dad to do so and sometimes refusing to get out of bed all day. It was making life difficult for us all, but especially for Dad whose social life was forcibly curtailed. We arranged carers so that Dad could go out but she got very angry and said that she wouldn't allow them in the house. One day I thought, 'Enough's enough.' I didn't shout at Mum but I just decided to take a stand. I told her that Dad was going out and that a carer would come to sit with her. When she started her usual tirade I just walked out of the room. I thought she would follow me and was prepared for trouble but in actual fact she just went very quiet. She accepted a carer after that and her anger was replaced by an occasional sulk, which I could deal with.

Don't allow the person with dementia to dictate to you or to the rest of the family. Try to work out which things really matter and make a stand over those things and those things only. Mostly these will be matters that concern the safety of the person with dementia or the safety of others. If the person with dementia wishes to drive the car when their licence has been revoked because they are considered unfit to drive, then you should take a firm stand and refuse to allow this. If the person with dementia wishes to pace around the garden in what you consider an aimless way, this may annoy you but it is not important. By trying to stop them you are increasing stress levels – and the possibility of an argument.

CONCLUSION

These tips should do much to help make life easier and less stressful for both you and the person with dementia. Many carers will not find it easy to adapt their behaviour to incorporate these suggestions , but if you can do this successfully you will go a long way to reducing the incidences of what mental health professionals like to call challenging behaviour (see chapter 4). So, in summary:

1. Accept that YOU need to change YOUR behaviour.
2. Do not ask complex questions.
3. Reduce the choices on offer.
4. Do not contradict.
5. Do not criticise.
6. Decide what is really important.
7. Do not let yourself be bullied or intimidated.

Chapter 7

Retaining independence

Early on, many people with dementia lose the ability to carry out everyday tasks or to keep going with a procedure and not be distracted. There are many ways carers can help them to continue to perform tasks for themselves without appearing bossy or interfering.

People with dementia gradually lose their ability to carry out everyday tasks. There are two elements to this loss. The area of the brain that governs 'executive' ability – that is, the ability to generate action – is often one of the first areas to deteriorate. This means that people with dementia find it very difficult to begin a task, even something quite simple such as washing hair or cleaning teeth. In addition, people with dementia seem to lose their 'procedural' memory early on, meaning that they find it difficult to carry out actions that involve following a sequence, including getting dressed or making a cup of tea, as well as more complicated tasks such as following a recipe or programming a washing machine.

Sometimes carers think that they can solve this problem by writing down the sequence of tasks for the person with dementia to refer to (for example, how to load and switch on the washing machine) and occasionally this works for a short while. Mostly, however, it does not help. The person with dementia is found to be unable to follow the written list. They may lose the ability to interpret what they read (although they may still be able to 'do the mechanics' of reading) and/or they may not recall where they are in the instructions at any given moment. Sometimes it seems that people with dementia just cannot begin to understand how to use the list to help themselves.

It can be hard for a carer to understand that certain tasks are, in fact, a series of actions, and they cannot understand why the person with dementia can no longer dress properly or butter a slice of bread. For his or her part, the person with dementia is often frustrated because he/she realises that they should be able to carry out certain tasks and they remember that they were able to do so in the past.

Sometimes people with dementia remember only the time when they could do these everyday tasks and, if you ask them about their day, they will describe what they used to do – getting up, making breakfast, catching the bus to the shops, doing the housework, etc – and not what they do now. They are not telling deliberate lies. Their memory no longer works in chronological order and they are recalling what they used to do as if it were the present day.

As explained in chapter 1 (page 10), there is no definite pattern to the deterioration in abilities. Although experts can now predict the general way in which dementia will progress, people do not lose their abilities in a particular order. It is possible for one person with dementia to be able to hold a good conversation but to need guiding into a chair or leading from room to room because their spatial awareness has disappeared. It is equally possible for someone else to retain the ability to play a piece of music on the piano but not to be able to hold a coherent conversation. Some people find their eyesight is badly affected by dementia (see page 117 in this chapter) and this will affect their capacity to carry out even simple tasks.

It is important that someone with dementia is encouraged to be as independent as possible for as long as possible: this will not only increase their self-respect, but will also make life easier for those around them and those involved in their care. There are many things you can do to encourage and help independence.

BREAKING DOWN TASKS INTO SIMPLE STEPS

It takes some thinking and planning to break tasks down into component parts. A classic example is the task of making a cup of tea, and this may be a good one to begin with if you are trying to work out how to plan the task. However, there are other actions of everyday living which you may consider more important. Let us look at getting dressed in the morning. This is something most of us do without thinking, apart from considering what clothes are appropriate for the day ahead. It can be disconcerting for carers to find that the person they are looking after finds the task difficult. Classic problems are:

- forgetting to remove night clothes before putting on day wear (and conversely forgetting to remove day clothes before donning nightwear)
- putting on two items of clothing – two shirts, two sweaters, two pairs of trousers or socks
- being unable to fasten buttons or zips
- putting clothes on back to front
- trying to put items of clothing on the wrong part of the body – putting arms into trouser legs, etc.

Not everyone makes all of these errors and not everyone makes mistakes all the time. As dementia progresses, more problems will be encountered more frequently.

Here's a logical breakdown of the steps involved in getting dressed:

1. Remove nightwear.
2. Choose clothes to be put on, in the right order – underwear first, for example.
3. Put the garments on – legs into trousers, arms into sleeves, and so on.
4. Fasten buttons and zips.
5. Select the next item.
6. Possibly we may need to change position – for example, we may need to sit down to put on socks or tights.

Here is how carers can help:
- Lay clothing out on the bed in the order in which it will be put on.
- Lay out only one garment of each type – one shirt, one jumper, one pair of socks etc .
- Keep the bed clear of any other items to avoid distraction.
- Take away any clothes that need washing so that they are not re-used.
- Be on hand to supervise discreetly and offer unobtrusive help.

Laying garments out in order helps the person with dementia to progress the task in the correct way. This will also ensure that only appropriate clothing for the season and activity is worn.

Keeping the bed clear of other items helps to prevent the person with dementia from becoming distracted. This is a common problem.

Laying out only one garment of each type keeps choice limited (see General behaviour tactics, page 101).

Removing dirty clothes before dressing commences prevents them being re-worn inadvertently.

The last point in the task list is important and applies to most tasks. As the disease progresses the person with dementia will need more and more supervision. Be sure to offer help in the most unobtrusive way you can. People with dementia are often acutely aware of their difficulties and get annoyed and frustrated when help is forced upon them when they feel (however mistakenly) that they do not need it.

You can chat quietly while handing clothes over one item at a time; or you can be 'occupied' in another part of the room and only step in to help when required. It is better not to intervene obviously by saying 'Let me help you with that' or 'You've done the buttons up wrong; let me do them' or by using any phrase that could be construed as criticism. If the person with dementia starts to put on the wrong garment or tries (for example) to put the wrong arm into the wrong sleeve, it is better to help them make the adjustment quietly and without comment.

If the person with dementia becomes angry and resents your help, go back to the point made in chapter 6 (General behaviour tactics, page 110) and decide whether the 'wrong' way of dressing really matters. If the person with dementia puts their sweater on the wrong way round or buttons up their shirt incorrectly, it doesn't really matter. You can leave things as they are if you are going to be at home all day. If you have to go out and you feel they need to be tidy, you can choose a moment later on to quietly correct the problem, perhaps re-doing the buttons while discussing the shopping trip or helping to remove the sweater 'because it will be too hot when wearing a coat' before you go out.

With a bit of practice you can break down any procedural task. Another example might be serving and eating breakfast. You can lay items of food and cutlery out in a clear and predictable manner and place each item on the table as it is needed. You might set the box of cereal out on the table for the person with dementia to help themselves and then remove it and replace it with the milk. After cereal has been eaten, take away the cereal bowl and lay out a plate with toast, setting butter and jam/marmalade nearby. Remember: if you are having to supervise diet (because of diabetes, for example) do not have 'forbidden' items in sight or on the table.

The key points to remember are: break the task down into simple steps; start the task off, perhaps with a gesture; give the person with dementia time; be clear what really matters in completing the task (such as safety issues); and stay on-hand unobtrusively in case help is needed to re-focus on the task.

Start people off on tasks

Some people with dementia find it difficult to begin an everyday task. This is often one of the early signs of dementia. Carers might say:

> *'She stands there helplessly looking at the bed as if she doesn't know what to do.'*
> *'He will wash his hands but neglect to dry them and come out of the bathroom dripping water everywhere.'*
> *'He puts his coffee cup on the table but doesn't seem to understand that he needs to pour coffee into it.'*
> *'She puts washing in the machine but forgets to turn it on.'*

People with dementia can often carry on with a task if you start them off. They might not be able to remember that they have to clean their teeth in the mornings, but if you put toothpaste on the brush and hand it to them they may well carry out the task successfully. Even at a much later stage in the disease, they may still be able to brush their teeth if you guide their hand with the toothbrush and help begin the action.

If someone doesn't seem to know how to prepare for bed and stands in the bedroom gazing around, begin helping them to take off their clothes and they may well continue the task. People often remember how to get into bed – the sight of the bed triggers that memory – but unless you assist them or guide them to undress, they may try to get into bed in their clothes, possibly even with their shoes on.

If you are doing a job such as sweeping up leaves in the

garden, you may find it puzzling and annoying that the person with dementia seems to stand around watching you helplessly. They are not being difficult. It is probable that they know they 'should' be doing something but they are not sure what or how they should start doing it. If you give them a broom and start them off with the action, they may well continue to sweep up leaves and even subsequently remember how to load them into a barrow and wheel it to the compost heap.

DIFFICULTIES WITH VISION

It is believed that up to 60 per cent of people with any form of dementia have impaired vision. It is important to understand what this means. Often when I suggest to carers that the person with dementia cannot see properly, they reply that they have already arranged an eye test and that the optometrist has said that there is nothing wrong. The first thing to understand is that we DO NOT see with our eyes, we see with our BRAIN. Our eyes just allow the light in; it is our brain that interprets what we see. Most people with dementia will have problems interpreting what they see at some point in the disease and for many this happens early on. Occasionally it is the first sign of dementia.

Many of the problems we encounter when we try to get people with dementia to follow a certain route, to sit in a place indicated to them, to go in the direction we are pointing, occur because the person with dementia has trouble seeing. Visual problems may also explain why many people with dementia stop enjoying hobbies such as reading, sewing or model making. These problems with vision of course, play a huge part in loss of orientation.

How to tell if there is a problem

It is not easy to ascertain whether someone with dementia can see properly. Normal eye tests may not reveal this, not least because someone with dementia may not be able to answer the optometrist's questions – for example, is the line darker against the red background or the green one? Nor can the person who has dementia easily explain their perception or lack of it. Occasionally someone with dementia states that they cannot see and is offered new glasses, magnifying lenses and large-print books. Often none of these is much help. It is really difficult to understand what problems someone with dementia is having because they have generally lost the ability to express what is happening or to explain what they do or do not see.

We do know that people with dementia often lose the ability to distinguish between blue and black. This can cause extra problems at dusk or when the light is failing. We also know that people with dementia have a problem with reduced contrast: this makes it harder for them to distinguish facial differences and recognise different people, among other things. We also know that people with Lewy body dementia have problems with patterns on floor and wall coverings so that they may see the patterns as differences in height and floor level. People with Lewy body dementia (and some other forms of dementia) may also see things which the rest of us cannot (so-called 'hallucinations').

It is probably best to assume that someone with dementia has some visual impairment or abnormal visual sense.

Look for clues

The behaviour of people with dementia can give you a clue. For example, if someone with dementia walks into a room and hovers about instead of sitting down when this is suggested, it is likely that they cannot see where the chairs are. It is no good pointing to a chair or indicating it with a wave of the hand. The best thing to do is to gently guide the person with dementia into the chair, letting them feel the back of the seat against their legs and staying by them until they are comfortable.

If someone with dementia ignores their cup of tea they may simply have forgotten about it. But, equally likely, they may be unable to see the cup; so pick the cup up and hand it to them or guide their hand towards the cup on the table so that they can feel for the handle.

Many people with dementia start to follow their carer around, which can be very annoying, but it may be due to difficulty in seeing where the carer is when they move away. One tip is to continue talking as you move out of view so that the person with dementia knows that you are still around.

Strategies at home and out and about

When someone with dementia says that they need the toilet, do not just point to the relevant door. Stand up with them and guide them into the toilet and make sure that they can see where the lavatory pan is before leaving them to it.

If the person you care for still likes to walk to the local shops alone, or take the dog out for exercise, it is good to encourage this. Be aware, however, that they may have limited vision and that if there is a change to the normal route (for example, if there are road works) or if something happens to cause them to be disorientated (such as meeting someone who stops to speak, perhaps causing them to turn in a different direction), then they may become confused and get upset and even lose their way.

In the home, try to keep cupboard contents and the layout of counter tops as consistent as possible and if you decide to move furniture around, take the time to show the person with dementia (probably several times) the new layout and allow them time to get used to it.

When you are out and about, do not leave the person with dementia alone without some point of reference. For example, you might say:

'I am just going to put this note in Mr Green's letter box. You stand here – here by the green gate – and wait for me. I am going up the path to his door and putting a note in the letter box. Wait for me here by the gate.'

Then, even if the person with dementia is no longer able to see where you are, they have the comfort of a fixed reference point (the green gate), which they can touch and know is there.

I must emphasise that the visual problems of dementia are not easy to understand. Each person is different because each brain is different and we should never assume that just because we can see something, other people can see it too.

There is more detail about visual problems with dementia in chapter 10 (see page 171).

Up to 60 per cent of people with dementia have problems with vision. These are problems with interpreting what the eyes transmit to the brain and will not show up in a regular eye test. Look for clues in how the person with dementia behaves and make sure surroundings are as consistent as possible so the person can find what is needed.

ENSURING THE PERSON YOU CARE FOR FEELS SECURE

As I have mentioned a number of times, many people with dementia start to follow their carer around and this can be very annoying to the carer. (See the tip above in 'looking for clues' and you may find this habit becomes less annoying.) This is often because they fear they will lose the person on whom they depend. You can sometimes help someone to feel secure by giving them a reference point (as in the green gate example above) or by giving the person with dementia something of yours to hold on to while you are out of sight – gloves or a scarf, for example. Sometimes you can give an 'alternative' source of security: for example:

>*'I am just going over to talk to Mary. John here will stay with*
>*you while I am talking to Mary.'*
>*'We are going into the bank now.'*
>*'We'll go into this cafe for a cup of coffee.'*
>*'I need to collect my coat from the dry-cleaner – just here.'*

If you meet someone when you are out, always remember to remind the person with dementia whom they are meeting as they may not recognise them immediately.

>*'Hello, Mike. Helen, it's Mike our next-door neighbour.'*
>*'Look, Mrs Johnson is waving at us. She works in the shop where*
>*we buy our paper.'*
>*'We are going to meet our son John in the tea shop – look there*
>*he is, waiting for us.'*

If you are helping someone with dementia to conduct some business, say in a shop or bank, avoid correcting them in public or making them feel stupid in front of others. Try gentle reminders to help them stay 'on track':

>*'Peter, weren't you going to ask for a new cheque book today?'*
>*'I think you were going to buy a new shirt. Shall we go and look*
>*at them over there?'*
>*'Can you reach a can of beans from this top shelf?'*

DON'T USE 'TEST' QUESTIONS

In my work I often meet carers who feel they are being helpful by giving clues or by asking 'test' questions. Look at the following examples:

'Who came to see us yesterday, John?'
'The man who helps us in the garden – do you remember his name?'
'We went to see our daughter today – who was with her?'
'We must go because we have an appointment. Do you remember where we are going, Peter?'

In actual fact this kind of clue-giving or prompting isn't really helpful. As previously discussed, questions only put the person with dementia under stress and this is not the way we would normally talk to our spouse or parent. It implies a teacher/pupil relationship and may even make some people with dementia feel as if they are back at school and being tested. It frequently makes them irritated, as well as frustrated if they cannot immediately find the answer. Some people will refuse to answer and the only response is a sulky silence. Others try to 'cover up' their problems with remembering by starting to talk around the subject. Here are some sample responses:

'Ah yes, yesterday. It was a very nice day. Very nice and sunny, a bit like today. Were you wearing your blue dress? It really was very warm...'
'We do have a man to help in the garden. It is a big garden – we cannot manage everything. Have you seen our garden?'

It is better and simpler to avoid prompting or testing and to simply state facts as you would to a young child whose understanding is limited.

'Our daughter, Susan, came to see us yesterday.' (Don't add 'Do you remember, John?')
'We have a man who helps in the garden. His name is Fred and you and he enjoy talking about the garden, John.' (Use a statement not a question.)

'We went to see our daughter, Mary, yesterday and her neighbour, Sally, was with her. Mary and Sally had a great chat about knitting patterns.'
'We have to go because we have an appointment. Peter is going to have his hearing aid checked.'

Give useful prompts

As dementia progresses it will no longer be enough to just start the person with dementia on a task. Short-term memory does not refer only to the remembering of facts – it also applies to remembering to take action and to continue to take action. So someone might pick up a cup of tea and take a sip when presented with the drink. However, if they put the cup down to allow the liquid to cool or to continue to take part in a conversation, they may well forget that the drink is there. On occasions like this it is worth offering gentle verbal prompts such as:

'Don't forget your tea.'
'Drink your tea now.'

Be careful, though, not to allow these prompts to begin to sound like commands – or the person with dementia will think you are 'ordering them around' or 'nagging', resulting in tension and stress. Keep your voice low and your tone neutral and try not to draw the attention of others to what is happening. Remember to allow the person with dementia time to notice for themselves – for example, sometimes just simply touching or indicating the cup may do the trick. Alternatively, you can offer a visual clue by picking up your own cup and drinking. Research shows that we tend to 'mirror' other people's movements and actions while having a conversation; if you pick your own cup up and take a drink the person with dementia may do likewise.

If you are leaving a person with dementia with another carer, such as a neighbour or friend, be sure to tell them if this sort of prompting is required. Otherwise, on your return they may say something like:

> 'I made her three cups of tea but I don't think she was thirsty because she just left them to go cold.'

Similarly, if someone with dementia is carrying out a task (such as sweeping up leaves), remember to give them prompts now and again.

> 'That's right, put the leaves in the barrow.'
> 'Let's sweep up this pile now.'
> 'We'll just clear this last pile and then we can stop.'
> 'Shall we put the barrow away now?'

People with dementia do not always completely lose their abilities to carry out a task and these simple reminders, prompts or talking through the steps of the task can help them to retain their abilities and independence – sometimes for a long period of time.

If you believe that the person you care for has forgotten how to do something, try starting them off on the task and you may be pleasantly surprised. Although you might think it's quicker to do it yourself, this helps neither you nor the person with dementia in the long run. Continuing to carry out everyday tasks and actions helps to retain the connections between the brain cells or neurons (it is sometimes called 'hard wiring' the brain). Although people with dementia seem to have a limited ability to learn anything new, encouraging them to continue to carry out simple tasks that they are used to will keep them functioning longer and will also make them feel useful and satisfied.

ALLOW EXTRA TIME FOR EVERYTHING

People with dementia need more time to do things. They need extra time to absorb a question or a situation, extra time to frame a sentence during conversation and extra time to carry out everyday tasks. They may need extra time to realise where they are when they wake up in the morning or when they get out of a car at the end of a journey (even a short one) – and to remember who they have come to see. If they are allowed the extra time in all these situations, many people with dementia can manage quite well. A carer who is impatient and gets irritated at this slowness may make the person with dementia feel useless and both of you may end up having an argument.

Life may slow down when you are caring for someone with dementia, but it can continue in a satisfactory way for much longer if you are prepared to allow this extra time. If you also remember to remind the person you are caring for at regular intervals, and in a non-confrontational way, what they are doing, you may find both of you are calmer and more satisfied with life.

Remember that the person with dementia will get satisfaction from carrying out tasks by themselves where this is still possible. Do not, for example, rush to button their coat or pull on their gloves if they can still do this for themselves. Allowing them to do so may take longer and you may sometimes feel embarrassed in front of others while you wait, but your own patience may inspire others and they too may learn to allow extra time and maintain the independence of the person who has dementia.

Recently dementia has been much more in the public eye and there is more awareness of the problems that people with dementia encounter – and more sympathy for and acceptance of the condition. Much effort is being put into creating 'dementia-friendly communities' (see Glossary) and to educate the general public, and this is very helpful. However, some generalised ignorance remains and it is important to help people understand that each person with dementia is an individual and that the form that their dementia takes is individual to them. It can be hard for someone who has no experience to understand that some people with dementia can continue to carry out everyday tasks (albeit perhaps more slowly) for a very long time; that others lose this ability early but may be able to understand and play a part in a good general conversation and that still others lose their orientation skills and may need to be guided to a chair or towards a doorway even though they can still read a book or a newspaper.

RESPITE

It is important to remember that, although the person you care for feels safe with you and often will not want to be parted from you, you too need some time to yourself. People with dementia are not able to understand this need any longer nor will they accept a reasoned argument that their carer 'needs a rest'. They are not able to realise that they are causing any stress and they are terrified of losing the person with whom they feel secure. (By the way, this does not always mean that they are kind and loving to their carer – often the opposite is true: see page 65.) Therefore anyone with dementia is likely to resist being separated from their main carer. They may make a huge fuss if the carer goes out alone, even if they are left with a 'substitute' carer, and they may refuse to attend a day centre or to even consider spending time in residential 'respite care'.

It may seem as if respite care has nothing to do with promoting independence. However, if you consider that regular and carefully planned respite will result in the person with dementia being able to remain longer in surroundings with which they are familiar – that is, their own home – then you will see that respite planning is all part of promoting independence as long as possible.

If you know the person with dementia well you will quickly

learn the best way to encourage and help them. If you don't know them well, remember the cardinal rule: **Give them time**.

CONCLUSION

As a carer you can enhance the independence of a person with dementia in many unobtrusive ways, including:
- breaking tasks down into simple steps
- being aware that there may be problems with vision and compensating for these
- ensuring the person with dementia feels secure
- not using test questions
- allowing extra time for EVERYTHING.

Chapter 8

Helping people with dementia manage everyday life

As the disease develops, people with dementia become less able to do the things they used to do with ease. We have already discussed the way that dementia develops at different rates and in different ways in each individual. However, there is a common trend in the loss of abilities, and to a certain extent this corresponds to the different 'stages' of dementia, though as I say throughout the book, the condition develops differently in each individual so the following is merely a general guide.

Early dementia – In so-called 'early dementia', there are clear-cut cognitive deficits on careful clinical interview. For example, there might be difficulty performing complex tasks, such as handling finances, or travelling. Denial is common. There may be withdrawal from challenging situations.

Moderate dementia – People with 'moderate dementia' will be unable to recall major relevant aspects of their current lives, such as an address or telephone number of many years, or the names of grandchildren. There will be some disorientation as to the date, day of the week, season, or to place. They will probably require little assistance with toileting, eating or dressing but may need help choosing appropriate clothing.

Moderately severe dementia – In 'moderately severe dementia' sufferers may occasionally forget the name of their spouse. They will be largely unaware of recent experiences and events in their lives. They will require assistance with basic activities of daily living and they may be incontinent of urine. Behavioural and psychological symptoms of dementia are common, such as delusions, repetitive behaviours and agitation.

Severe dementia – In reaching this stage, sufferers will have lost their verbal abilities – that is, their ability to use words. They also lose their ability to walk. They will be doubly incontinent and need assistance with feeding.

As I explained in chapter 1, these stages are not definitive and it is sometimes possible for someone with quite advanced dementia to carry out activities that most others at that stage of the disease cannot. Conversely, some people may lose some abilities at a much earlier stage.

There is a fine balance to be struck in helping someone with dementia keep active and independent. It is beneficial for them to do as much as possible, but carers should avoid being too 'managing'. Boredom can be a major problem so it is worth finding activities that will keep this at bay, including making positive use of a day centre.

IN THE EARLY STAGES

At the onset of dementia, pre-diagnosis even, people tend to be defensive about their difficulties and memory problems, possibly denying them altogether, or at least making light of them and attributing them either to natural causes (*'Everyone forgets things as they get older'*) or to the failings of other people (*'You make me so flustered'*; *'You're telling lies about me'*).

Chapter 8

They generally try to behave as 'normally' as possible and feel threatened by any suggestion that they have any problems or even by close association with people who are further down the disease path than they are. Thus they may resist going to doctor's appointments, refuse the help of any support worker and avoid and speak rudely about people around them who have a diagnosis and show signs of dementia. Generally, people at this stage of dementia can still care for themselves, although sometimes they may need prompting. If they maintain a strict routine they can often continue to live an independent life, although they will begin to forget appointments, names and sometimes what they were doing. People at this early stage may resent the well-meaning attempts of family and friends to help them and may alienate their close friends, neighbours and family by their behaviour. Spouses and close partners of people who are at this stage may be bewildered by what they see as a 'personality change' and may consider breaking up the relationship until they realise what is behind the difficult behaviour.

At this stage people may stop some of their normal activities and hobbies, especially if these involve them in making decisions, becoming involved in complicated arrangements, or remembering a series of things (see page 6). They may feel less confident and begin to avoid actions or places that make them feel 'unsafe'. Close partners may notice that hobbies that involve the person with dementia in taking the initiative (organising a fishing trip, arranging a tennis match) are no longer happening. The person concerned is unlikely to admit to this, usually stating that they are 'taking a breather' or 'going to arrange a trip next week'. Indeed, in their own mind it is probable that at this stage in the development of dementia they really do intend to take action at some unspecified time in the future. They are unlikely to have made a conscious decision to 'give up' their hobby or undertaking but find the organisation required to take action just too difficult 'at the moment'.

131

Sometimes a minor injury or a short spell in hospital may be a big enough disruption to routine to make it difficult for the person at this stage of dementia to pick up their activities where they left off. Hobbies and pastimes that involve a friend or partner may be maintained for much longer as long as the other party makes all the arrangements or encourages the person with dementia to continue to participate. So, for example, husbands and wives who have always gone walking together may continue to do so and mothers and daughters who have enjoyed a weekly shopping jaunt may keep this up for quite a while.

Those who accept support manage better

It is unfortunate that people who could gain a great deal at this stage in the disease by accepting just a very small amount of help are the most reluctant to do so.

I tried to keep up my husband's interest in gardening because I knew he had enjoyed it in the past. Unfortunately, whenever I suggested a spot of gardening I was accused of 'nagging' and it caused a row. In the end, I employed a gardener and I thought he would protest a lot but he barely acknowledged what had happened.

I wanted my Mum to live as independently as possible. When she started neglecting the housework I thought it would help if we got someone to come in and help clean once a week. She was furious and accused me of interfering in her life. She wouldn't let the cleaner past the door.

At this stage of the disease people can often carry on with their normal activities, such as simple shopping, housework, gardening, reading newspapers and books, watching television and visiting the cinema, if they can get help when needed. Many also carry on with volunteering activities, although those who work with them may realise the problem and may need to offer extra help or unobtrusively lighten their duties. People at this early stage of dementia who are still in employment may begin to get into trouble at work because they find themselves in a muddle, unable to meet deadlines or carry out some tasks.

Employers who are unaware of the problem may begin to give warnings or to institute management supervision, resulting in premature retirement. Occasionally, occupational health may be involved and at this stage the diagnosis may be made.

People who are living with a partner who is able to support them may continue to manage many activities, although the partner may find him/herself helping them to do so.

Stepping up your involvement

A key indication that someone may be developing dementia is the loss of the ability to manage everyday finances. Often, someone who has always managed the household money begins to forget to pay bills, to ignore important documents like tax returns or vehicle licence reminders, or omits to check bank statements when previously they would have been meticulous about these matters. In households where one person has always dealt with all financial matters, the first sign of these difficulties may be when a utility is cut off because bill reminders have been ignored or when police stop someone who discovers that they have been driving without insurance. This can be a big shock to those who have always assumed that financial matters were being handled well. Situations like this tend to happen where one person in a partnership deals with all money matters and does not allow the other partner to become involved. Where both people in a partnership manage the money together, then the person who has dementia may begin to allow their partner to gradually assume responsibility (often on the excuse that they 'do not have time' or are 'busy at the moment') and over a period of time they opt out of managing the finances altogether.

> *My husband had always managed the money. It was pure luck that one day I found a 'final demand' for the electricity bill on the very day the power was due to be cut off. I managed to make a telephone call to the power company and get an electronic payment put through for the bill, but it was a shock to realise how close we came to being cut off. My husband seemed quite unconcerned and even got cross when I tried to point out what had happened. I manage the money now.*

Think about important financial matters

If you are caring for someone who is the usual manager of financial affairs in your household, do not assume that they will continue to control this aspect. It is important that you begin as soon as possible to handle things jointly, to find out where important documents are kept and to ensure that you see copies of bank statements, for example, and have knowledge of vital passwords for electronic banking and bill paying and that you take over bank cards and get PIN numbers issued in your own name. You should not delay doing this because you do not wish to upset the person with dementia. They may be resistant but you could explain that you need to know 'just in case anything happens to you'. Some carers find that they can gradually move bills and so forth into their own name without making a big issue of the matter; for others it is more difficult. This is a vital area of life and failure to pay mortgages, utility bills and legal items, such as vehicle licences, can result in real difficulties. HM

Revenue and Customs can sometimes be understanding, but utility companies are often less so and the police have a statutory duty to prosecute in certain matters. For example, it is your duty to ensure that your vehicle is insured and you cannot claim that you thought your partner had dealt with the matter and expect not to be fined.

Carers of people at this early stage of dementia can best help by encouraging them to continue their usual activities as much as possible, including hobbies and social commitments. This may mean that you will have to take over or help with some of the practical arrangements. Try not to become too 'managing' as you may be accused of 'nagging', and the person you care for may refuse to take part.

If you can make meetings and social occasions seem spontaneous, so much the better. You may find that if you make arrangements too far ahead and warn the person with dementia about them beforehand, they become apprehensive and refuse to take part. Remember that any social occasion (even an enjoyable one with friends) becomes stressful for someone with dementia and they may not look forward to it as they did previously. Short-term memory problems also mean that the person you are caring for may forget about a future event but may still recall a feeling of uneasiness that was evoked when you talked about it. They cannot remember what is to going happen on a certain day, but they will remember that they are apprehensive about it. It's best not to give too many warnings about upcoming events and not to discuss even pleasurable activities too far in advance.

BOREDOM AS THE DISEASE PROGRESSES

As the disease progresses people with dementia become less able to enjoy things they used to like doing. They will probably find it difficult to concentrate. It becomes hard to follow the plot of a film or television programme. However, many people do continue to enjoy watching moving images on the TV even after they are no longer able to understand the story line. Enjoyable programmes include nature documentaries, where the commentary is secondary to the images, sports coverage, if the person with dementia enjoyed sport previously, and 'niche' programmes, such as films about steam railways or sailing ships or craft and cookery programmes – again these will continue to be enjoyed if it was a previous interest or hobby.

Sometimes people with dementia (usually in the later stages but it can happen earlier) become confused and afraid of images on TV – especially news items about war or disasters. They may believe the events are happening right there and that the pictures are of a scene just outside. Some people start to believe that newscasters or commentators are talking directly to them and they may become frightened, either because they do not know the person on the screen or because they do not understand what they are being told. If this happens, it is best to leave the television turned off as the person with dementia may become very agitated and it will be hard to convince them that what they've seen is on the TV rather than all around them.

Although many people with dementia retain the ability to read, they may be unable to recall what they have read previously – even one or two sentences ago – and this makes reading a book stressful. They may just stop reading books but still continue to flick through a newspaper or magazine and enjoy the 'normality' of doing so. Sometimes people will read a newspaper over and over again, forgetting that they have previously read it. If this happens there is no need to comment upon it or to stop them. The person you care for is getting the same amount of enjoyment from the sixth time of reading the newspaper as from the first time – they do not remember reading it before.

You could look out for books that do not require great concentration or use of memory. Books with plenty of photographs, such as travel books, nature books and local history, or 'souvenir' books about current or historical events, are ideal. These books do not require so much concentration and nor does the reader need to hold in their memory what they've just read. Family photograph albums are also often enjoyed at this stage. If your photos are stored on your computer, print them off and make them into an album that can be enjoyed from the comfort of an armchair, rather than getting the person you care for to stare at a screen.

Keeping boredom at bay

When people become less able to concentrate or remember enough information to allow them to enjoy their usual leisure activities, they may quickly become bored. Many carers don't realise that boredom is a significant factor in difficult behaviour. Someone who is bored may fall asleep easily, may become restless and pace around, may get agitated by small things or may begin to indulge in anti-social activity (for example, masturbating in public or shouting and swearing at others). It can be difficult to find things to entertain people at this stage because there are very few things that they can continue to do without some supervision.

Outdoor activities

Where the person you care for can still be trusted to find their way around, asking them to do simple outdoor activities ensures that they get fresh air and exercise. Examples include walking to the shop for the daily paper or walking the dog, sweeping up leaves in the garden, taking the rubbish out to the dustbin and mowing the lawn. Some people can continue to do routine chores like this with minimum supervision and will enjoy an activity which makes them feel useful. Keep things simple: asking a person with dementia to shop for several items may not always be successful even with a list, but collecting the newspaper is straightforward, especially if they've always done this.

The person with dementia may still enjoy bystander activities, such as watching a football match or other sporting event, a parade or carnival, or grandchildren acting in the school play, but it is best if you accompany them to events like this in case they forget why they are there and become confused.

Most women and some men enjoy continuing to carry out household tasks, such as peeling vegetables, vacuuming the floors, folding or hanging out washing, ironing and dusting. Anyone doing these tasks may still need to be supervised, but this can be done from a distance and sometimes with only minimum intervention. For example, whilst you are cutting sandwiches for lunch the person with dementia may set the table, get out the plates and cups or mugs for tea and so on. Many women with dementia seem to enjoy ironing and can continue to do it safely and well, especially if this was something which they liked and did often previously. Both women and men may enjoy folding linen (men seem less keen on ironing!) and towels and pairing socks is a simple task which needs little supervision.

Using domestic appliances

Sometimes at an early stage, and often later, people with any form of dementia find it more difficult to operate domestic appliances, such as washing machines, dishwashers, microwaves and remote control units for TV and hi-fi. Carers sometimes think that they can write some simple instructions to prompt them, but often this does not seem to help. When appliances break down or become worn out and have to be replaced, this usually creates difficulties. New appliances are seldom the same as those they replace and the person with dementia is unlikely to be able to learn to operate them. People living alone may become unable to cook because they cannot learn how to use a new cooker or microwave machine. Sometimes this precipitates the employment of a care agency whose workers will be able to help provide a cooked meal among other things.

It is better if carers understand that they will probably be unable to teach the person with dementia to operate any new appliance and also if they understand and accept that the ability to use even familiar appliances will gradually fade away. This saves extra stress to both carer and the person with dementia – for the carer, the stress of trying to teach 'new tricks', and for the person with dementia, the stress of the natural annoyance and exasperation of their carer.

Therapeutic activities

Some people with dementia continue to enjoy gardening, particularly if this was a favourite hobby. However, carers are likely to discover that gardening is a more complex business than it at first appears. Simple routine jobs, such as sweeping up leaves or mowing the lawn, can often be continued, but the person with dementia may lose their ability to distinguish between weeds and seedlings or to tackle more complex jobs, such as pruning or planting out. This doesn't mean that they won't enjoy their time in the garden, and men who spent time pottering in their sheds may continue to do so quite happily, although they will gradually achieve less and less. (Some wives may claim they don't notice much difference!)

Dementia can make people anxious and so even those who previously spent hours alone in the garden may begin to feel agitated unless they can see the person who cares for them. Gardening is thought to be therapeutic and many community efforts are made to set up 'dementia-friendly' or 'age-friendly' garden spaces.

My husband enjoyed working on his allotment for many years and when he first developed dementia he continued to visit the allotment every day when he could. At first I think he managed pretty well and we still had many vegetables for the table but, over time, although he continued the routine of 'going to the allotment' I discovered that he did less and less actual work. One of our neighbours eventually told me that he was spending most of his time wandering aimlessly around and sometimes even lost the way to his own plot. Because I seldom went along to the allotment it was quite a while before I found this out, but when I did I felt we had to give the plot up for someone who could make more use of it. The local council don't like it if you don't keep your plot cultivated. I think my husband missed the routine more than anything else and he often got very restless about the time he would usually have gone over there.

Walking for pleasure can be enjoyed for a considerable time as long as the person with dementia has no disability which prevents this. Walking is also known to be an excellent form of exercise. Carers often worry about risks, such as crossing roads, but people with dementia may retain their innate reflexes and ability to negotiate traffic for quite a long time. If you are the main carer you should be aware of the possibility that the sight of the person you care for has deteriorated (see chapter 7, page 117); check periodically that they can still see traffic and other obstacles clearly, or more to the point, understand what they are seeing. If someone is prone to falls it is obviously not sensible to allow them to walk alone regularly – neither is it a good idea if you feel that they might lose their way when out alone.

Becoming lost even in familiar surroundings may sometimes be a problem: refer back to chapter 4 (page 58) for tips on how to cope with this.

Indoor activities

A person with dementia who enjoyed jigsaw puzzles may well be able to continue doing them long after they can no longer look after themselves. Keen knitters may also be able to carry on knitting – although they may no longer be able to follow a knitting pattern. Someone may enjoy playing a musical instrument long after their ability to read music has passed. Where the brain has been, as it were, 'hard wired' or 'programmed' to carry out an activity, the ability to do so can continue for longer than we might expect.

Don't get fixated on the notion that the person you care for (or, indeed, you) needs to do crossword puzzles, brain-teasing games and sudoku to keep the brain active. What is important is to give the brain new experiences and opportunities. Many people with dementia still enjoy going to exhibitions, outings and visits, and although they are usually less able to learn new things or to enjoy new activities, as I've explained, they can be encouraged to keep up with things they have always enjoyed.

USING A DAY CENTRE

Many carers flinch away from taking the person they look after to a day centre, perhaps because of an old-fashioned idea that it is somewhere where people are 'dumped' to be out of the way – kept warm, sheltered and fed, but not stimulated or entertained in any way. They feel they are 'failing' if they place the person they care for in a day-care facility and that they should shoulder the burden of care themselves; if they ask others to help, they are showing a lack of love for the person they care about, and in addition, accepting a day-centre place acknowledges the decline of the person they care for.

Some carers worry about how to persuade the person they care for to attend the day centre, especially as, in the early stages of the disease, people with dementia often refuse to go, particularly if they see others there whose illness is more advanced than their own. Other carers are certain that the person they care for will really dislike the day centre. They see it with their own eyes as a place full of people with needs, a place where activities may sometimes seem childish or patronising. They are unable to picture that, for someone with dementia, the day centre may be a place of safety and comfort, where no unnecessary demands are made and where others understand their predicament.

> *It was quite difficult at first to keep insisting that my husband attend the day centre, but the staff encouraged me to persist. He cannot tell me what he does there or whether he has enjoyed himself. All I can say is that on his 'day centre' days he is quite different. When he comes home he is more settled – tired, I think but more contented – than on days when we spend all day at home together.*

Good day care includes stimulatory experiences for the person with dementia. To the carer, looking on, some of the activities may seem patronising, even infantile, but they are seeing these activities through their eyes, not through the eyes of the person with dementia. Handicrafts, board games and quizzes may seem childish activities, but someone with dementia may find them challenging, enjoyable and fulfilling. I have seen a scientist who previously headed a research department thoroughly engrossed in a quiz at the day centre. I have watched senior engineers enjoying card games, chefs enjoying cooking simple biscuits, teachers taking part in flower-arranging – all of them enjoying every minute. I have seen ex-senior civil servants taking great pleasure in watching a train set running.

Even those who shun the activities on offer enjoy the company of undemanding companions and the conversation they get from their peers. Many people with dementia who do not want to take part in activities enjoy watching others do so. At the day centre someone with dementia can enjoy watching birds around a bird feeder, can help to plant out seedlings in the garden, can just sit in the garden and enjoy nature without feeling under any pressure.

Good day care also incorporates reminiscence, both in structured sessions – where people gather to look at items or pictures from the past and discuss them – or by using visual, auditory and tactile aids. For example, a day centre may have an 'office' area with an old typewriter, paper files and hole punches and caddies full of pens and pencils. People who worked in an office in the past may linger in this area enjoying the familiarity of the items around them. The day centre might have a 'workshop' area or a 'shed' with pieces of timber, nails, screws and tools, and some people might enjoy the familiarity of this. Of course, in order to provide these experiences there must be good supervision and a high level of well-trained staff. There might be a room where different types of music can be enjoyed or where old posters and advertisements and news cuttings can be displayed . There may be various areas where items like jigsaw puzzles or handicrafts or painting can be enjoyed.

I hope this makes you, the carer, think about investigating the day-care facilities on offer in your area. You will have to pay for the person you care for to attend the centre unless your income is very low, but you'll find it is well worth it. If you are still undecided, consider this typical exchange at a memory clinic where the wife of a man with dementia is questioning the point of her husband attending a day centre.

> Psychiatrist: *'I understand you have been attending the day centre, Mr C. How is that going?'*
> Mrs C: *'There isn't much point in him going really. He doesn't do anything there.'*
> Care worker: *'Actually, Mrs C, he takes part in quite a few activities. The thing is that people with dementia often don't remember what they have been doing all day.'*
> Daughter: *'We discussed this, Mum. It's a good thing for you*

*because you get a break and it is a good thing for Dad because
he gets to see people and take part in things.'*
Mrs C: *'But if he doesn't do anything is there any point?'*
Psychiatrist: *'He clearly does take part in activities. As the care
worker has just explained, he just doesn't remember them.
Mr C, do you enjoy the day centre?'*
Mr C: *'It's fine.'*
Mrs C: *'But if he doesn't do anything why make him go?'*

Settling in at the day centre

At first people with dementia may resist the idea of going to a day
centre and for the first couple of visits they may be unenthusias-
tic. New situations are stressful for them; they will have to meet
new people in different surroundings from those they are used to
and they won't have the security of their carer being with them.
However, as they become familiar with going to the day centre,
they will be able to relax. The staff are all trained in dementia
care and are accustomed to helping people with dementia. As
they settle in at the day centre, the person with dementia will
begin to feel that he or she is accepted for what they are and for
what they are capable of. They will not be subjected to the stress
of managing situations that are difficult for them. After a few
visits, people who are able to express an opinion usually say that
they enjoy their time there and look forward to going.

*'I don't know how often I go to the day centre now. All I can tell
you is that when the bus turns up at the door I'll happily get on
it and I don't worry about what is going to happen there.'*
'I can be myself.'
'I don't have to worry for the whole day.'
'There is always someone to talk to.'
*'I am friendly with a couple of the other chaps there and we have
a good laugh.'*

Chapter 8

> *'The other ladies and I often talk about our grandchildren. It doesn't matter if we can't remember their names.'*
> *'The staff are so friendly and I don't feel as if I'm being "kept up to the mark" like at home.'*

The 'mid-stage' of dementia can be the toughest time for carers and day care can make a real difference. A good day centre may continue to look after a person with dementia even after they move into a later stage of the illness (see below).

ACTIVITIES FOR THE LATER STAGES OF DEMENTIA

As dementia progresses people may constantly bang their hands on the chair arms, shout or swear, sing at inappropriate moments and be generally restless. People become less able to speak or communicate and definitely less able to understand speech.

Some carers continue to manage to care for the person at home, usually with additional help in the form of agency carers.

Although there are fewer activities for them to enjoy because of their reduced capabilities, people with dementia still continue to enjoy being entertained, although they may fall asleep more often and have a shorter attention span. They often continue to enjoy having poetry read to them. This may sound strange as we may think that a level of intellectual ability is required for poetry comprehension, but poetry is essentially rhythmic and appeals to the emotions.

People in the later stages of dementia often still enjoy taking part in singing groups and other musical activities for the same reason. Songs and poems from the past may be remembered with real pleasure and often people who can no longer speak easily can still sing the words of a favourite song. They may also enjoy watching other people taking part in activities. For example, someone at this stage of dementia may no longer be able to take part in cooking or flower-arranging, but they may enjoy watching others carry out these activities.

At home, even someone at an advanced stage of dementia can enjoy watching 'the world go by', so seating them by a window or in an area of the house where people are coming and going may be beneficial. They can still enjoy the natural surroundings of a garden or a park or beach – watching birds and small animals, feeling the breeze on their skin and the sun's warmth. Some people still enjoy television and films at this stage, simply watching the movement and colour on the screen. Others find moving images too distracting and even frightening, but it is worth experimenting.

Stroking the fur on a soft toy, handling a piece of velvet or running the hands over a piece of smooth wood are examples of pleasant tactile sensory experiences that some people with dementia enjoy. They often carry out an activity like this in a compulsive way that they clearly find satisfying but that can annoy you, the carer. Try to focus on the pleasure that is gained by the person with dementia and forget your irritation: compulsive stroking movements are not harmful and may be soothing.

Clearly there are now few activities that the person with dementia can enjoy alone, so this is a good time for you to call on your 'team' (see chapter 2) for help. Explain clearly to your team members what you'd like them to do.

If it is possible to arrange it, physical exercise is still beneficial. Some people will still be able to enjoy walking, dancing and possibly swimming if carefully supervised. For people who are less mobile there are chair exercises. Look out for 'dancing for health' classes arranged by local authority community centres and by Alzheimer Society day centres. It is tempting to leave someone sitting in their chair for long periods if they seem contented and express no desire to move about, but this is not a good idea. Muscles become lazy from lack of use and stiffen up, and physical exercise can help improve sleeping patterns and appetite.

Chapter 8

In the very late stages of dementia the person with the disease becomes less and less responsive. They may become unable to move voluntarily and may keep their eyes closed most of the time. Carers can still stroke their hands, talk softly, perhaps recite poetry and play music or sing to them quietly.

Chapter 9

Lifestyle

Is there anything that can be done to help slow the progress of dementia in the person you are caring for? Medication may be appropriate and research shows there are lifestyle changes that are well worth trying.

Although we still do not know precisely what causes dementia and we still do not have a definitive cure, we do know that there are some steps that may help to slow down the progress of the disease. These are generally lifestyle changes, which are also thought to help to prevent dementia developing in the first place. The medical professionals you meet may be sceptical about some self-help methods, but you have nothing to lose by helping the person you care for to make simple adjustments to their lifestyle, improve their diet and follow simple strategies to make the most of the times you have together.

A word about medication

Medications can improve symptoms, or temporarily slow down the progression of the disease in some people. As I describe in chapter 1, there is evidence that two classes of drug – cholinesterase inhibitors and NMDA antagonists (see page 16) – may help some people with Alzheimer's disease, improving their motivation, anxiety levels, confidence, memory and general mental abilities. These drugs may possibly also help people with dementia with Lewy bodies, but there is little evidence that they help those with vascular dementia.

After a diagnosis, you and the person you care for should consider accepting any medication you are offered, at least for a trial period. Many people are put off by the mention of side-effects. Modern-day protocols mean that doctors have to point out the possible side-effects of any drug they prescribe. This does not necessarily mean that the person you care for will experience these. Medications come with an explanatory leaflet which details possible side-effects and also the likelihood of these occurring. If 10 per cent of people are likely to have side-effects, this means that 10 out of every 100 people who take the drug will suffer them. It also means (perhaps more importantly) that 90 out of every 100 people who take the drug will NOT suffer side-effects. Most of the dementia drugs are given at a lower dose first, partly to allow for monitoring of side-effects. Your doctor should explain this to you and should try to ensure that the person with dementia understands so that they can make a considered decision.

The reason for at least trying out medication is that, limited in effect as these drugs are, they are the best solution that medicine can offer at the present time. Remember that dementia is progressive; it does not go away or get better on its own. If the person you care for refuses dementia drugs they are refusing the medical treatment that is available. If they do suffer from side-effects, these may only last for a short time, or the doctor may be able to adjust the dose to minimise them. If the worst comes to the worst, the patient can stop taking the medication but it is still worth giving it a try.

Not everyone can be offered the medication that is available as there are some contra-indications (health reasons why someone should not take the medicine). Your doctor will explain these to you if they apply. If he/she does not explain this, you and the person you care for should ask why they are not being prescribed medication. Since most of the dementia drugs are now 'off licence' they are comparatively cheap and should be freely available where there is no medical reason to indicate otherwise.

People with dementia are, of course, under no obligation to accept drug treatment and suggesting that it is worth a try does not take away the individual right of choice in this matter. Carers may need to remember that the decision to take or not take medication is really a decision for the person with dementia.

Practically speaking, most people with dementia will need help to remember to take any medication and so if you are their carer you need to keep in mind that you should act always in their best interests and consider what they themselves would want rather than your own feelings.

Helping yourself – lifestyle changes

People who cannot be prescribed 'memory drugs', and even those who are taking them, will often ask what they can personally do to help themselves. Sometimes doctors are not very helpful at discussing non-medication solutions, but this is an area where a dementia support worker, or dementia adviser, can be very helpful.

There are four main lifestyle areas (exercise, nutrition, socialising, and using the brain to work things out or consider new things) where self-help is useful. People with dementia may not be able to understand the need to alter their lifestyle – or they may be less able to make the changes that can help. As a carer, you can take the lead in these areas and do your best to help – it may not always be easy but it can be worthwhile.

Exercise

There is a large body of evidence from research studies that suggests physical exercise both prevents the onset of dementia and slows the progression of the disease in people who are already showing symptoms. If you would like to read more about some of this research for yourself, then chapter 5 in my book *The Essential Guide to Avoiding Dementia* is a useful resource.

Exercise is known to have many positive effects in all older adults, including those with disabilities. In particular, it prevents or reduces the risk of problems that occur as a result of limited movement (often referred to as a sedentary lifestyle), such as coronary heart disease. The beneficial effects of exercise on the heart and the blood vessels – the cardiovascular system – include stimulating the supply of blood to the brain. A better supply of blood to the brain will prevent or decrease damage to the brain.

Exercise is worthwhile even after memory problems have become obvious. Alzheimer's disease and other dementias are linked to a more general physical deterioration. People with dementia are more likely to show signs of under-nutrition, to have a higher risk of falls (and consequent broken bones) and a more rapid decline in mobility than would be expected through normal ageing. Improving the physical condition of people with dementia may extend their independent mobility and their quality of life.

With an appropriate exercise programme even quite elderly people with dementia can improve their cardiovascular function, their ability to use their muscles easily and without pain, their balance and their strength. Anyone who improves their flex-ibility and balance is less likely to fall over, so reducing the risk of injury or admission to hospital. A severe fall may result in a bad loss of confidence for someone with dementia, making them more dependent on you, the carer, and less likely to try activities on their own. So you can see the value of exercise for anyone with dementia.

If you are caring for someone with dementia you may think it will be impossible to get them to an exercise class. However, exercise can take many forms and any exercise is better than none at all. You can encourage the person you are caring for to move about more, you can suggest and join in with a regular walk. You will always have more success if you encourage them to carry on with something they've enjoyed in the past, rather than trying to get them to try something new. You can encourage and help the person with dementia to continue any hobby which involves physical movement – for example, gardening, bowls, golf or yoga. You might need to register the person you care for at classes, remind them of the golf club hours, perhaps drive them to the venue where classes or fixtures take place, and ensure that they have the relevant clothing and equipment.

How to overcome resistance to exercise

You may encounter resistance from the person with dementia, due in part to a condition that doctors call 'vascular apathy'. This means that people with dementia tend to lose their 'get up and go' and are unable to motivate themselves. When this happens it is time to enlist your 'team' members (see chapter 2) to help. A friend who has always attended the same golf club or yoga class or bowls club could call round and accompany the person you care for. Look out too for 'walking for health' groups that you can join together – these are often advertised on the noticeboard at your GP's surgery or in the local newspaper. Remember walking is good exercise for both of you.

Gardening is a form of exercise too and you can encourage the person you care for by doing jobs together – even if previously you haven't done much gardening. If you engage a professional carer to keep the person with dementia company and provide some respite for you, then the carer will be happy for you to suggest activities they can do together, such as walking or following an active hobby, and this would be a good use of their time and your money.

There are some people with dementia who become restless and seem to have a compulsion to walk around – sometimes not stopping to sit down and rest at all during their waking hours. Others grow restless and start to walk around only at certain times of the day (see chapter 4). Although we do not know why people have this compulsive urge to walk around, it has been found that regular exercise planned and organised during the day can have a good effect on mood and may reduce the amount of seemingly 'aimless' walking. If the person you care for becomes restless at certain times of the day, it may be worth re-arranging your combined schedule to make that the time for exercise. It is possible that restlessness and compulsive walking, while sometimes annoying to the carer, may be simply the body's way of encouraging activity – which is actually beneficial. So consider whether you really need to stop the person you care for acting in this way. Perhaps if the person you care for wants to go out for a walk it may be better to allow this, going with them if you fear they may get lost or fall over.

Exercise in the later stages of dementia
As dementia progresses, some people become more frail and less fit generally. Sometimes the affected areas of the brain include those that control movement, the limbs and gait. There are many walking aids available to help those who become less mobile and at any stage in the illness you can ask for an assessment by an occupational therapist to see if a walking aid will help. If the person you care for has frequent falls, then ask for a referral to the local 'falls team' for advice (see chapter 3, page 40) about ways to avoid falling over and relevant balancing aids.

Even if the person you care for is becoming less mobile, try to encourage them to move around frequently. This may mean simply moving from room to room or from bed to chair – even these simple movements will help with circulation. Some local authority leisure centres offer chair exercise sessions – exercises designed to be done sitting down.

Physical exercise has proven benefits for someone with

dementia. If you want to help slow the progress of dementia then encourage exercise and help to make it happen.

Nutrition

Diet is one area where you can really help the person you are caring for. Someone with dementia is suffering from a serious illness and they need optimum nutrition to help their body to function as well as it can.

Everyone has their own ideas about a good diet and there are a number of research trials which involve different foods or food supplements. It is now known that there is a clear link between type 2 ('maturity onset' – meaning that it develops in older people) diabetes and dementia, and that type 2 diabetes is also linked to a large intake of refined carbohydrates and obesity. Many people with dementia develop a craving for sugar even in the early stages of the disease. The brain needs glucose to function properly and it is possible that the body is reacting to the brain's reduced ability to process and use glucose by craving a higher intake of sweet foods. Of course, because the brain is less able to process glucose, eating more sugary foods will not be helpful and you should try to limit these. (For more on diabetes, see chapter 10, page 167.)

Dementia may also affect the sense of taste and smell, and some people with dementia lose their appetite or change their eating habits quite early in the disease, so it is important to be aware of this. Someone who has a reduced sense of taste or smell will benefit from more highly spiced food, perhaps with more added salt than you would normally use, even though this may go against what you have been told is 'healthy'. To help with loss of appetite try giving smaller meals at slightly more frequent intervals.

'What should I cook for the person I care for?'
As I have said, diet is one area where you can really help the

person you are caring for by providing optimum nutrition to help their body to function as well as it can. You should switch to using 'whole' unrefined foods where possible if you do not already do so, and avoid processed foods and those containing unnecessary additives. Use wholemeal bread, brown rice and pasta, rather than white refined versions. Use whole (full-fat) milk, butter (not low-fat 'spreads') and full-fat cheese. If you are having to supervise diet (because of diabetes, for example), do not have 'forbidden' items in sight or on the table.

Reducing sugary foods. In this respect it is worth remembering that fruit is rich in fructose – which is sugar by another name – so don't overdo fruit in the diet. Although some fruits (citrus fruits, kiwi fruit) are a good source of vitamin C, many vegetables are just as good. Increase servings of vegetables – but don't overcook them and remember some can be served raw in salads.

You may think that since the brain needs glucose to function, reducing sugar intake is an odd suggestion. However, the body converts starches to sugar so any starchy foods or carbohydrates – including brown rice, pasta and bread – will be converted into the glucose that the brain needs. By serving unrefined carbohydrates you will be ensuring that the body has a steady intake of glucose rather than the 'rush' of sugar that the brain experiences after eating high-sugar foods, such as cake and biscuits.

'The person I care for keeps forgetting to eat'

If you are caring for someone who lives alone they may forget to eat at all – or they may forget that they have eaten and eat one meal after another. Often, the part of the brain that 'switches off' appetite when the stomach is full does not work properly. A 'meals on wheels' service can be ideal for people living alone – then at least you can be sure they have one meal each day delivered ready to eat.

Another solution is to arrange for an agency carer to call in at lunch or dinner time to ensure that a meal is prepared and eaten.

You can also invite the person with dementia out for meals or cook for them regularly at your home. Arranging a place at a day centre will also help as this normally includes a meal as well as refreshments throughout the day.

You can offer to shop or help with the shopping for someone living alone to make sure that they have enough food in the house. This will also let you check that food is not kept beyond its 'use by' date and also to see whether the person with dementia is still able to manage simple cooking safely. Such steps may be helpful if someone is living alone and is in the early stages of the disease, but as the dementia progresses it is unlikely that the person you care for will be able to carry on living on their own as, along with other loss of ability, they will almost certainly become unable to cook safely or to manage their own food intake.

'Should we try food supplements?'

Some recent research has indicated that people with dementia may benefit from certain food supplements. The evidence is not conclusive, but there is nothing to be lost by trying out a supplement provided the person you care for takes the recommended dose. For details of the research into various supplements you can read chapter 6 in my book *The Essential Guide to Avoiding Dementia*.

Foods which seem to help some people are:

Coconut oil – This has been promoted heavily in the USA and some trials are currently underway to try to establish whether it really does help.

Turmeric – There has been some research into the potential role of turmeric as a treatment for Alzheimer's disease, and there is anecdotal evidence of its benefits. Most research is centred around curcumin, a chemical found in turmeric.

B vitamins (especially folic acid) – Supplements may help people where their level of vitamin B complex is low; once again, the evidence as to its use as a treatment for dementia is not conclusive.

Vitamin D – Many elderly people have low levels of vitamin D. The best way to obtain this is to expose the skin to sunshine (although you should follow guidelines about sun exposure) during the summer. In the winter the sun in the UK/northern Europe is not strong enough to produce much benefit so some people like to take a supplement.

Doctors rather frown on any suggestion of taking supplements or cooking with special foods, such as coconut oil or turmeric, but in the recommended amounts these are unlikely to do any harm and may be of some benefit. Most people would be prepared to try anything to help themselves and most carers would do the same to help the person they are looking after. However, beware of claims made for expensive food supplements which claim to be 'dementia foods'. There is no real evidence to show that these do any good. If you read the ingredients, you may find that you can get the same benefit from a simple multi-vitamin or supermarket buy.

'The person I care for is losing weight'

Weight loss is quite common in people with dementia. It can happen early on in the disease, possibly even before diagnosis. It often happens with other serious diseases too, such as cancer, and it isn't always possible to pinpoint the cause. The person losing weight may appear to eat normally and to enjoy their food.

Other people with dementia begin to lose weight at a later stage in the disease. If this happens, you should take even more care to ensure that everything they eat is as nutritious as possible. Ignore current health guidelines about low-fat diets. Use full-fat

milk on cereal, porridge or in drinks, full-fat cheese in sandwiches and recipes, and avoid anything labelled 'low-fat'. Eggs
are an excellent food for someone with a poor appetite; they can
be cooked in so many different ways, are extremely nutritious,
and easy to eat. Eggs can be eaten every day (ignore past health
guidelines about eggs raising fat or cholesterol levels – these are
now thought to have been wrong).

Nutritional problems that develop later in the illness
'The person I care for has lost his/her appetite'
If the person you care for seems to lose interest in food later in
the illness, when previously their appetite has been good, then
you should take notice. Sometimes people with dementia develop difficulty in swallowing. You may notice that they chew
food for a long time or that they cannot swallow pills easily. They
may start to refuse food for this reason. If you suspect the person
you care for has difficulty swallowing, ask the GP for a referral
to the speech and language therapy (SALT) swallowing service
for an assessment. The therapists will be able to advise about
food preparation and other ways to help the person you care for.
People with advanced dementia may not be able to explain they
have a problem that makes eating difficult: for example, tooth-
ache, ill-fitting dentures or mouth ulcers. A dentist may be able
to pinpoint and help with these problems, but, as the carer, you
need to be alert and try to spot if the person you care for seems
to be in pain or discomfort when eating.

'The person I care for ignores his/her meals'
Sometimes, as the disease progresses, people with dementia simply 'forget' to eat. The solution may be as simple as reminding
them that the food is there and sitting with them to ensure they
do not wander away from a meal due to loss of concentration.
Some people with dementia may forget how to use a knife and
fork, for example, or how to drink from a cup. Various eating and

drinking aids – such as lipped plates and special cups – are available and may help at first, particularly if the problem is a lack of co-ordination or spatial problems; however, later in the illness some people may have to be spoon fed. If the person you care for attends a day centre, the staff there should be able to cope with any of these problems.

Carry on socialising

There is considerable evidence that points to the benefit of good social networks, satisfying interaction with others and a feeling of being useful, in helping people to remain fit and healthy into old age and in avoiding the symptoms of dementia. At the most basic level, a good social life can help people stay aware of the date and time – all useful practice for getting to appointments and meeting up with friends. However, the importance of social interaction goes beyond this basic level. Meeting and talking to other people stimulates the brain and gives us new experiences and new thoughts. Just as our bodies need exercise to stay fit, so our brains need stimulation to remain active and flexible.

When considering brain stimulation, it is important not to get fixated on the notion that it is necessary to do crossword puzzles, brain-teasing games and activities like suduko to keep the brain active. What is important is to give the brain new experiences and opportunities to develop. This need not be difficult. Many people enjoy going to exhibitions, on outings and on visits. Many people continue to study new subjects as they grow older. Others enjoy taking up a new pastime or sport. All these things stimulate the brain. People with dementia are usually less able to learn new things or to enjoy new activities, but they can be encouraged to keep up with things they have always enjoyed and to participate in activities or hobbies they are familiar with.

'We've always kept ourselves to ourselves'

When I support people with dementia I often hear the words, 'We are just not sociable people'. Well, of course, it is your right not to be sociable and I'm not suggesting that people who have always been quiet and retiring need to force themselves to become 'party animals'. What I would suggest is that most of us gain something from interaction with others.

If you are caring for someone with dementia, it is likely that they may have become more withdrawn and less sociable even before the diagnosis. This is because as the disease progresses it becomes harder for the brain to cope with new and potentially stressful situations. In addition, as has previously been pointed out, one of the first symptoms of dementia is the loss of the 'executive function' which causes one to get up and do things. You as the carer can help. While you should not force someone to take part in any activity or to go out and meet friends, you can encourage, coax and assist them to do so. The place to start is activities they have enjoyed in the past (see chapter 8, page 139 for tips). Day centres also play an important part in socialising (see chapter 8, page 141).

Chapter 10

Health

Modern medicine has encouraged us to believe that there is a 'pill for every ill' – and where we cannot cure a disease, in many cases we can control it or relieve the symptoms, so that we can lead a normal life. It can therefore come as a shock to learn that the medication available to help in cases of dementia is very limited.

Drugs to treat dementia

Medical treatment (where available) varies according to the type of dementia – one reason why early diagnosis is so important. It can relieve symptoms or temporarily slow down the progression of the disease in some people. (For details of drugs available, see chapter 1, page 16.)

After the diagnosis, the person you care for should consider accepting any medication offered – at least for a trial period. See chapter 9 for full discussion of this subject.

Seeing beyond dementia

When someone has been diagnosed with dementia it often seems to those around them that doctors are unable to see beyond the dementia. Sometimes carers say that they find it difficult to get the GP to take symptoms of illness seriously and that they are dismissed as being 'part of the dementia'. Family and friends may also dismiss symptoms of other illnesses as due to dementia. However, people with dementia are as likely as anyone else to suffer from minor and major illnesses, and since any illness or discomfort may make the dementia temporarily worse and the person with dementia more confused it is important that illness is addressed promptly. Colds, chest infections and urinary infections are just as likely to occur in someone with dementia as in anyone else. People with dementia may also suffer from other conditions such as arthritis, diabetes, poor eyesight and hearing problems.

Visiting the GP

Many things can make it difficult for someone with dementia to have a satisfactory consultation with their GP. Because of confidentiality issues, some GPs insist on seeing the person with dementia alone and this can lead to real difficulties since the person with dementia may forget why they are seeing the doctor or may not be able to explain symptoms clearly. Occasionally the person with dementia is the one who insists on a consultation in private. In either of these two cases, it is likely that the person with dementia will forget what the doctor has said or be unable to convey the doctor's advice to the carer. As the carer, you should try to accompany the person with dementia into the consulting room. If this is not possible, then write a note to the doctor setting out the reasons for the appointment and drop this off at the surgery before the consultation. Reception staff at the surgery will usually help you with this.

Communication between the GP and the person with dementia during a consultation is also likely to be difficult. GPs who are not familiar with dealing with dementia patients may ask questions that the person with dementia cannot answer such as: 'How often do you feel sick?' Or the GP may take replies too literally. Asked about pain, a person with dementia may deny feeling pain at all if they are not experiencing it at that precise moment. They will be unable to remember that their leg (for example) was painful yesterday or is always painful when they walk.

Someone with dementia may even deny that they have had a fall because they cannot remember the incident. In these situations, carers should make sure that they present the doctor with the correct facts, even if this risks annoying the person they care for.

CLUES TO ILLNESS

As the carer and chief person in the life of the person with dementia, you need to keep an eye out for health problems. There are some medical conditions that affect elderly people in particular, and the sooner they are recognised and treated, the better. Because people with dementia may not be able to communicate easily and tell you if they are in pain or feel ill, symptoms can be missed. This section is not supposed to replace qualified medical help and advice, but is intended to help you as the carer to make a decision to call for the doctor when necessary.

What to look for if someone has had a stroke

Strokes are not always dramatic. A stroke may be so mild that it goes almost unnoticed. There are two kinds. Put simply, one is caused by a 'bleed' in the brain and this type of stroke may come on gradually. If he/she is able to explain, the person you care for may complain of an intense headache that is not relieved by normal painkillers. He/she may start to move very slowly, to slur their words and to be unable to understand what you say to them. They may vomit.

The second type of stroke is caused by a blood clot that prevents blood reaching a part of the brain. This is likely to be more sudden in onset. The person you care for may stop moving or speaking suddenly, they may fall down, their face may distort downwards on one side and they may lose the use of the arm and leg on one side. They may lose consciousness. With any of these signs call the doctor immediately.

A less easily recognised stroke might be so mild that the person you care for simply says they feel tired or dizzy; they may say that their arm or leg feels heavy or that they have tingling or 'pins and needles' in the limb. They may not be able to tell you any of these things but you may notice them moving with difficulty, becoming more confused than usual or failing to use a hand or arm, or perhaps walking with a limp.

Subtle signs to be alert for are:

- difficulty speaking or speech that does not make sense
- complaints of heavy or tingling limbs on one side of the body
- inability to use an arm or leg in the usual way (for example, the person with dementia may just use one hand and a fork when normally they would use a knife and fork properly)
- drooping on one side of the face
- Sudden inability to make sense of things that are said to them
- headache that is not relieved by normal pain killers
- loss of balance.

People who suffer a mild stroke may recover completely in a few hours or days, or they may have slight but permanent damage, such as a weak hand grasp or a leg that drags slightly when walking. When multiple strokes happen, the damage may get worse and remain worse with each stroke. However, there is no set pattern and someone may make a very good recovery from a second stroke after making only a slow recovery from the first one.

If you suspect even a mild stroke, it is essential to call the doctor. Prompt treatment is known to improve the chances of recovery. When someone has dementia it may be difficult to distinguish a stroke from normal slowness and confusion. You should take notice if the person you care for acts differently than usual or seems much worse in their confusion.

Diabetes

Diabetes is a serious condition that can lead to other health problems. Symptoms that might indicate diabetes include:
- passing urine more often than usual, especially at night
- increased thirst
- extreme tiredness
- unexplained weight loss
- genital itching or regular episodes of thrush
- slow healing of cuts and wounds
- blurred vision.

If the person with dementia begins to suffer from these symptoms, arrange for them to see the GP as soon as possible.

Someone with dementia who also has diabetes is likely to be less able to control their own blood sugar levels, to take their medication or to be aware that they need to eat or take medication at certain times of day. Wide variations in blood sugar may make dementia symptoms appear worse. If possible, as carer, you should take over monitoring the person's diet and medication, and make sure you are familiar with the signs that someone's blood sugar is too low.

Urinary tract infections

Urinary tract infections (UTIs) are common and seem to be more so in older people – although no one is sure why. They are also more common in women than in men. They can usually be easily treated with a course of antibiotics.

A UTI can cause someone to become severely confused. This can be frightening for the carer if they don't realise what is causing the change in behaviour. You should suspect a UTI or other infection in someone who otherwise appears well (but see symptoms below) and who shows a sudden increase in confusion and agitation – or who starts to experience hallucinations. Doctors may refer to this as 'acute confusional state' or 'delirium', and it can develop over one or two days. When someone who has dementia suddenly appears much more confused, their family and carers may be taken aback by changes in their behaviour and believe that the dementia is suddenly becoming worse.

Someone with a UTI may feel:

- pain or a burning sensation when urinating
- a need to urinate often
- pain in the lower abdomen (tummy).

Infections can occur in the upper or lower urinary tract. The lower urinary tract refers to the urethra – the tube that carries urine from the bladder to the outside of the body – and the bladder. The upper urinary tract includes the kidneys and infection here is potentially more serious.

Symptoms of a **lower UTI** include:

- cloudy urine
- needing to urinate more often during the day or night, or both
- pain or discomfort when urinating
- an urgent need to go to the toilet
- urine that smells unusually unpleasant
- blood in the urine
- pain in the abdomen
- back pain
- a general sense of feeling unwell.

Chapter 10

Symptoms of an **upper UTI** include:
- a high temperature or fever of 38°C (100.4°F) or above
- uncontrollable shivering
- nausea
- vomiting
- diarrhoea
- pain in the side, back or groin that is often worse when urinating.

Any of these symptoms can make real difficulties for someone with dementia because they may not understand what is happening and they are likely to be unable to communicate how they are feeling.

Always seek medical help if you see a sudden change in behaviour. Normally a urine specimen will be needed to check whether there is an infection. It can save time to take a urine specimen into the surgery for testing before making an appointment with the GP or practice nurse – especially if the person you care for has had a UTI previously and you recognise the symptoms. You can buy kits that help you to take urine specimens from incontinence pads if necessary; ask your district nurse (or local continence adviser, if there is one) for advice and help.

If there is an infection, a course of antibiotics will alleviate the symptoms. You can help by encouraging the person you care for to drink plenty of fluids and take any medication properly. When the person with dementia recovers from the UTI, their additional confusion and agitation should disappear.

Colds, flu and chest infections

People with dementia are as likely to catch a cold or 'flu as anyone else. As the carer, you should keep in mind that any infection can make someone with dementia more agitated, confused and upset. If the person you are caring for becomes more agitated and their moods seem to change for no apparent reason, you might suspect that they are going down with an infection and – unless it is obviously a common cold – arrange an appointment with the GP to have it checked out.

Bear in mind that the immune system of someone with dementia is compromised – that is, it isn't working as well as it should at fighting off infection. Every effort should be made to protect someone with dementia from catching infections, even a common cold, and especially chest infections. Discourage friends and family with coughs and colds from visiting someone with dementia, be careful about hygiene if you have a cold yourself, and do not take the person you care for to the day centre if they are not completely well.

COPING WITH PAIN

Someone with dementia may not complain of pain. There is a common misconception that people with dementia do not feel pain, but this is not true at all. Short-term memory loss means that someone who suffers from intermittent pain may not re-member this when questioned. So, for example, if they suffer pain at night (as is common with some forms of arthritis), they may not remember this and may say that they have no pain when questioned during the day. It is also possible that, as the disease progresses, the concept of the word 'pain' becomes harder to understand and so someone with dementia may not be able to answer if you ask them whether they are in pain.

There are some obvious clues that the person you are caring for is in pain. He/she may:
- avoid using the body part that hurts
- groan or cry out when moving a painful body part
- refuse to get out of bed or stand up from a chair
- rub or clutch the affected body part
- refuse to eat (which may indicate mouth pain)

- be unusually confused or agitated when asked to move about
- contort their face into an expression of pain when moving.

If you need to ask someone with dementia about pain you may need to be specific. In the early stages of dementia it may work to ask simply, 'Where does it hurt?', but as the illness progresses you may have to use a process of elimination. For example, you could touch each arm or leg and ask 'Does it hurt?' Touching the body part will help to draw attention to the area. This will be far more effective than asking 'Does your left leg hurt?' Avoid generic questions such as 'Do you have any pain?', which will be difficult for the person with dementia to interpret and respond to.

If the person you are caring for is a regular sufferer from a painful condition such as migraine or gout, you will already be aware of this and familiar with the symptoms that indicate an attack. You can then administer medication, or contact the GP if required, in good time to avoid severe pain.

If there is no other explanation – such as an infection (see above) – for agitated or difficult behaviour, then consider the possibility of pain before asking the doctor or perhaps the dentist for further advice.

DEALING WITH HALLUCINATIONS

Most people with dementia have visual problems. Sometimes these are very obvious: someone with Lewy body dementia, for example, may have vivid hallucinations – which to them are very real. They may see people, animals or objects and they may find these hallucinations frightening or agitating. People with Lewy body dementia may also have problems in interpreting what they see, with judging distances and with perceiving objects in three dimensions. If you are caring for someone with Lewy body dementia you can get further advice from a dementia support worker (if you have one), a community psychiatric nurse or from online factsheets such as those provided by the Alzheimer's Society.

The best way to manage these hallucinations is to acknowledge that the person with dementia can see them, but not to give them too much attention. It does little good and may greatly upset the person with dementia if you insist on telling them that the people or things that they see do not exist. For example, if the person with dementia is seeing dogs and asks, '*Are those dogs yours?*' you can simply answer '*No. They are not mine,*' rather than saying '*There are no dogs – you're seeing things.*'

If the hallucinations are very upsetting and the person you care for becomes agitated, it can help to say something soothing such as, '*They will go away in a moment if you sit quietly and ignore them*', or '*We won't take any notice of them tonight.*'

Lewy body dementia is not the only form of dementia to affect the eyesight. It is difficult to know exactly how someone's vision is affected because the person with dementia cannot usually tell us. Even an eye specialist may be unable to tell exactly – see chapter 7, page 117 for more information. However, as far as possible you should still try to make sure that the person you care for continues to have normal eye tests and checks because any extra problems, such as short-sightedness or distorted vision because of the wrong spectacle prescription, will make things even more difficult. If the person with dementia wears reading glasses, try to make sure he/she continues to use them.

LOSS OF HEARING

Hearing impairment generally happens as we get older and people with dementia are no exception to this. Research published in 1989 found that untreated hearing problems were more common in those with dementia and that the risk of dementia increased with the degree of hearing loss. The researchers did point out that there was no suggestion that hearing loss was a cause of dementia; rather that hearing loss might make symptoms of dementia more obvious or that someone with dementia might have more significant symptoms because hearing loss increased their difficulties generally. When someone can't hear properly they can become isolated – unable to join in conversations or to understand what's going on. Ultimately this can contribute to depression.[1]

As communication is vitally important for someone with dementia, you should make every effort to detect hearing loss and to get help with the problem. A person who has dementia who also has a severe hearing loss will be likely to be more confused if they cannot hear what is going on around them. People with dementia are often reluctant to wear hearing aids, even when they have been prescribed, and carers sometimes find it difficult to ensure that they are worn consistently.

If the person you are caring for was used to wearing hearing aids before their diagnosis, they will probably be able to use them independently for a while, but they may not realise when they need cleaning or when the batteries are low. As the carer, you will have to be vigilant about this. Try keeping a note of how long the batteries last, and how often the aids need cleaning, so that you have something to refer to when the person you care for is no longer able to let you know. Many local community hospitals have a 'walk-in' service for hearing-aid adjustment and cleaning, and for new batteries.

When you visit the memory clinic with the person you care for, there is a special version of the memory test that can be used for people with hearing problems. Notify the clinic in advance if you would like this test to be used as the doctor or nurse may not always have this version with them.

1 Uhlmann Richard F, et.al. Relationship of Hearing Impairment to dementia and Cognitive Dysfunction in Older Adults. (1989) *JAMA* Vol 261 no 13. 1916-1919.

Ensure that everything is done to improve the ability of the person with dementia to hear. At home, keep background noise, such as the radio or TV, to a minimum. Do not talk across the TV or radio – switch it off while you are speaking. Face the person you are talking to and raise your voice if necessary. Do not allow others to carry on background conversations while the person with dementia is trying to speak or listen. When you are out and about, use touch to attract the attention of the person with dementia, so that he/she can face you to speak and listen.

ROUTINE HEALTH CHECKS

People with dementia often handle routine health checks, such as visits to the optician, the dentist or the hearing clinic, without any problem. These appointments may actually be less stressful for them than a visit to the memory clinic. This is because a dental appointment, while not necessarily pleasant, is something they have encountered before – something routine.

In the early stages of dementia, health checks may present few problems. However, if you are caring for someone with dementia you should try if possible to be present for these checks as you may be able to explain symptoms on behalf of the person you care for and perhaps to interpret their replies to questions. It is very important that health professionals take extra care to use their powers of observation with people who have dementia, rather than simply relying on replies to any questions.

Dental care is important to ensure that problems are dealt with in good time. A tooth abscess or severe tooth decay may cause extreme pain and result in more confusion, distress, anger and even violent reaction in someone who has no concept of time when waiting for pain relief to work. The dentist can advise you how to help the person you care for clean their teeth when they become unable to. They may suggest the the person with dementia lies down and you approach from behind the head to clean their teeth. However, a person with dementia may not tolerate this. Whatever you do, remember to tell the person you are caring for what you are doing and to KEEP repeating this to reassure them – it can be very unpleasant to have your teeth cleaned by another person.

There are dentists who are trained specifically to treat people with learning needs and now that 'dementia-friendly communities' are becoming fashionable, there are several dentists who have experience at looking after people with dementia.

Someone who has a dental plate or false teeth may refuse to wear it in the later stages of dementia. At an earlier stage in the disease, some people lose their sense of acceptable behaviour and remove false teeth in public and show them to others, as if they no longer understand what they are used for (as indeed they do not). This can be gently discouraged by the carer. If this kind of behaviour becomes a severe problem, you could consider helping the person with dementia to wear their false teeth only when they actually need them to eat.

At the opticians/optometrist the carer may need to help interpret replies to questions as well as explain from their own observation any problems the person with dementia may be having. As already explained, people with dementia may have visual problems that cannot be corrected with spectacles and it is important that you understand this and don't just think the optometrist is not doing his/her job properly.

Other health appointments, such as visits to an outpatient's clinic or for a blood test, are often taken in their stride by people with dementia in the early stages. However, someone with dementia may find it difficult to wait their turn or to take a place in a queue. Try to arrange plenty of distraction and reassurance while you are waiting. Remember that, as always, you may need to remind someone with dementia constantly about where they are, why they are waiting and why they are seeing the doctor. For procedures such as blood tests and blood pressure readings, take the time to explain to the person with dementia what is happening.

> 'The doctor is going to test your blood pressure (indicate the equipment)... Let me help you roll up your sleeve... put your arm on the desk... the doctor is testing your blood pressure... keep still... he is checking your blood pressure. Now you can roll your sleeve down.'

Some doctors are very good at reassuring a person with dementia; others are not so good, so be prepared to help. Do not be embarrassed at intervening. The well-being of the person you are caring for is your responsibility and the doctor should understand this and be glad of your assistance. If the doctor insists on seeing the person with dementia alone, try explaining why you need to be there.

> 'I won't interfere, doctor, but my husband/wife will be happier if I stay.'
>
> 'My mother will not be able to understand your questions. I can help explain to her.'

Someone with dementia may still experience other health problems, both minor and major. It is important to keep any regular health checks up to date. Do not assume that every health problem is due to dementia, but do remember that dementia is a debilitating illness and that any other minor infection or illness may cause the symptoms to worsen temporarily. It is also worth remembering that not all the health professionals you encounter will be familiar with dementia. You may well know more about how to manage the person you care for than the health professional concerned.

Chapter 11

Practical matters

When someone you love has just been faced with a diagnosis of dementia, it is likely that practical matters concerning the future come to the forefront of your mind. Things that many people avoid thinking about, such as making a Will, granting Lasting Power of Attorney or choosing a care home, now assume much more significance.

It is very important not to put off dealing with practical matters. Lasting Power of Attorney, Advance Statements, Advance Decisions and making a Will can only be done when the person with dementia still has the mental capacity to do so. Likewise putting claims for benefits in place and planning for care home fees are much more easily done when the person with dementia can contribute, though the carer will need to shoulder the administrative burden.

PLANNING FOR THE FUTURE

One of the objectives in the government's push for earlier diagnosis of dementia is that this gives people who have dementia more time to make decisions about their future care. As the disease progresses, people with dementia become less able to do this. They may not understand the points they have to consider. They may be unable to marshal their thoughts sufficiently to come to a considered decision. They may not be able to 'argue their case' with their relatives and carers. Even if they have strong feelings about their future, they will become gradually less able to express them.

As a carer, you can help in these early stages. It is often difficult for someone even in the early stages of dementia to take action. They may cover up this inability by saying that they are considering the matter, they intend to look at it tomorrow, they don't want to be rushed, and so on. It is a genuine kindness and is acting in their best interests for the carer to move things along, to send off for forms, to complete them, to help the person with dementia to understand them and to encourage them to sign where necessary. This is not to suggest that someone with dementia should be left out of the decision-making process if they are still capable of being involved. It is meant to encourage you, as the carer, to go ahead and begin sometimes tedious and bureaucratic procedures and to make things easy for the person with dementia.

Let's look at these important matters individually.

Note on country-specific information: My experience of dementia care has been entirely in England, so the details of information below relates to England and Wales. However, the PRINCIPLES of what needs to be addressed and when will be equally true for anyone caring for a person with dementia.

ATTENDANCE ALLOWANCE AND RELATED BENEFITS

Attendance Allowance is a payment given to someone who needs extra help – literally, someone to 'attend' to their needs. At the time of writing most people with dementia will be entitled to receive Attendance Allowance. It is not 'means tested' so you do not have to declare your income on the application. The form asks very specific questions about what the person applying for the allowance is able to do – for example, there are questions about bathing, dressing, preparing food and so on. One section of the form covers things like confusion, inability to understand letters and forms and to communicate.

There are two levels of allowance. The lower level is granted for people who need help only during the day and the higher level for those who also need a high level of care at night. If the lower level is granted initially and later you feel that the higher level is needed, you can apply for the higher level at that stage.

Attendance Allowance is currently under discussion and there is a suggestion that it might be replaced by a grant to local authorities which would allow them to give grants where they feel money would be most useful – in other words, the allowance would depend upon the rules of the individual local authority.

You can download the forms to apply for Attendance Allowance from https://www.gov.uk/attendance-allowance/how-to-claim or get them by telephoning the number on that site (0345 605 6055 at the time of writing) and asking for them to be posted to you.

It is a good idea for carers to complete the forms without consulting the person with dementia. This may sound very wrong but the questions on the form are quite intrusive and personal. The person with dementia may become upset if they have to answer them and they may deny that they are unable to do some things (such as wash and dress themselves). My experience is that people with dementia (and some carers) tend to make light of any problems they are having, with the result that the grant of Attendance Allowance may be refused when it should not be. It is a good idea to ask a support worker or an adviser to help you complete the forms objectively. Alzheimer's Society workers, Carers' Support Workers and Citizens' Advice Bureaux advisers will all be able to help you.

Council Tax Disregard

People with dementia who are in receipt of Attendance Allowance are also entitled to apply for Council Tax Disregard. This is not the same as Council Tax Benefit – literally, the people with dementia will be 'disregarded' when council tax is assessed. This usually means a 25 per cent reduction in council tax or (if the person lives alone) they will no longer have to pay council tax. Council Tax Disregard needs to be applied for on forms supplied by your local authority – look on their website, or telephone or call at the council offices to get the forms.

CARER'S ALLOWANCE

This may relate to you, the carer. Carer's Allowance is for people who regularly spend at least 35 hours a week caring for someone with a disability who him/herself receives a Disability Living Allowance (Middle or Higher Rate for Personal Care), Attendance Allowance or Constant Attendance Allowance (paid as an addition to a War Disablement Pension or Industrial Disablement Benefit).

To receive the allowance (which is taxable), carers must not be in full-time education or earning above a certain amount. You must also be living in the UK when you claim the allowance.

The person you are caring for may lose some of the benefit they receive (for example, a severe disability addition), as a result of the carer's allowance claim so you need to check this out. Usually this only applies if the disabled person lives on their own and does not include underlying entitlement awards of Carer's Allowance (see below).

You cannot receive both Carer's Allowance and a State Retirement Pension, so many carers of someone who has dementia will not qualify. If, however, you are a carer who would otherwise qualify for Carer's Allowance, you may be entitled to what is known as Underlying Entitlement, which may in turn entitle you to other benefits.

Some people may be entitled to other benefits and allowances, such as Mobility Allowance, Personal Independence Payments, Pension Credit, winter fuel payments and 'blue badge' parking permits. The benefits system is complicated and not every detail can be covered in this book. The Citizens' Advice Bureaux (CAB) give excellent advice about benefits of all kinds and they have a useful website which helps you work out whether it is worth applying (see reference section). You can also get more information on the www.gov.uk website.

Being in receipt of certain benefits often qualifies you for other financial help or gives you priority when claiming 'non-cash' benefits (see Underlying Entitlement above). Some benefits are means tested and the entitlement may in itself mean very little. You may think that, say 40p a week, is not worth the effort of claiming, but the extra benefits to which it may entitle you, or the person you care for, may make it worthwhile.

PLANNING FOR CARE HOME FEES

If the time comes to consider moving to a residential care home or a nursing home, the person you care for may not meet the criteria for state financial assistance for care/nursing home fees, or they may choose to enter a care home independently of any state aid.

If the local authority is involved in arranging your placement, the amount you will have to pay will be worked out via a means test, which is based on nationally set guidelines.

At the moment, your capital and savings below £14,250 are disregarded in the means test. If you have between £14,250 and £23,250 in capital and savings and your need for care reaches the threshold set by your local authority, then the council will subsidise your care costs according to a sliding scale.

The government is making changes to the funding of long-term care as a result of the Dilnot Commission (July 2011) and, as part of these changes, the government will set out national 'eligibility criteria' that will apply to everyone, wherever they live. This means that the current rules will change.

Paying for care is a complex subject, and everyone's situation is different. You should seek advice about your individual case. There are organisations which offer specialist advice about this. The social care team will be able to advise you about your eligibility for state financial assistance and will carry out a financial assessment of your case if you request this.

See the reference section for details of useful sources of up-to-date information.

LASTING POWER OF ATTORNEY (LPA)

Lasting Power of Attorney (LPA) is a legal process in which someone, in this case the person with dementia (referred to in 'legal language' as the 'donor'), hands over to someone else (the 'attorney') the power to manage their finances and property and/or their health and welfare if it becomes necessary.

It is always a good idea for the person with dementia to give Lasting Power of Attorney to someone (or several people) they trust.

Many people put off doing this, but Lasting Power of Attorney can only be given when the 'donor' has the mental capacity to understand what they are doing, so it is best to do it as soon as possible. If the person with dementia is unable (because they lack mental capacity) to give Lasting Power of Attorney, no one can do so on their behalf and instead a complicated application to the Court of Protection (see below) is required.

The diagnosis of dementia does not in itself mean that someone is no longer able to make a Lasting Power of Attorney. The person with dementia must be able to understand what it means, and many people in the early stages are perfectly able to understand this, even if they find it difficult to complete the relevant forms. It is vital to help them organise Lasting Power of Attorney as soon as possible after diagnosis.

As their carer, it is likely that the person you care for will want you to be an attorney for them, but they may prefer to appoint someone else (a son or daughter, for example). They can appoint more than one attorney and this may be a good idea as the attorneys can then share the work involved. It can, however, make difficulties if more than one person has to sign every cheque or letter to the bank, so this does need thinking about.

You can fill in the forms to apply for an LPA online at the government website gov.uk (see reference section for full details). This is by far the easiest way to do it if you are comfortable with filling in forms online, as there is no risk of muddling up sheets of paper – especially if you are applying for both types of LPA at once (see below) – and getting them in the wrong order. If you prefer you can print off the forms and fill them in by hand. If you don't have a computer or access to the internet, you can ring up the Office of the Public Guardian (see below) and request the forms plus an information pack to guide you through them (see reference section, page 211, for phone number). There is no need to use a solicitor to help you apply for a Lasting Power of Attorney.

Once you have filled in the forms and got them signed and witnessed (this process is explained in detail on the website and in the printed guidelines), you must register the LPA with the Office of the Public Guardian (see below) before you can start acting as an attorney.

(Note: There is a different process in Scotland and Northern Ireland.)

LPA for property and finance

Having this LPA means that you will be able to help the person with dementia pay their bills, use their bank account, claim benefits and manage their pension, for example. You may need to help them pay for care and may eventually have to help them sell their house. Once the LPA is registered (see below) you can start helping straight away. If you discuss finances with the person with dementia as soon as possible, you can build up a picture of how they manage their money – how much birthday money they like to give their grandchildren, how much money they spend on clothes, which charities they like to give to, and so on. Ask them to show you where they file bank statements, bills and so forth. In that way you will then be in a good position to take over when they can no longer manage their financial affairs.

LPA for health and welfare

Unlike the property and finance LPA, once the health and welfare LPA has been registered (see below), you cannot start using it until the person with dementia has lost the capacity to make their own decisions. In the meantime, talk to the person with dementia and make notes: you could discuss any medical treatments that they may or may not want, where they would like to live if they have to move, what they want to happen to their dog or cat if they can no longer look after them, and so on. Once they have lost the capacity to make decisions, you will have to do it for them and if you have gained a good sense of what they like and dislike, you will be able to make decisions that are in their best interests.

Registering an LPA

The person with dementia or the person who will be their attorney must register the LPA with the Office of the Public Guardian. This process can take up to 14 weeks – another reason to get started before the situation is urgent. There will be a fee to register each LPA, which is reduced if the person with dementia has a limited income and savings.

If the LPA is accepted, the Office of the Public Guardian will return the original document to you with each page stamped and validated. The registered LPA is a valuable document – keep it somewhere safe. If you lose it, the OPG will issue a copy for a fee.

Making certified copies of an LPA

Banks, building societies, utility companies, and so forth, may all want to see a copy of the finance and property LPA. Doctors, care homes, social workers and others may want to see a copy of the health and welfare LPA. To avoid losing track of the original documents, you need to get some certified copies made – simple photocopies will not be accepted.

The person with dementia can make their own certified copies if they are still able to write and to understand what they're doing. It involves photocopying the document and writing and signing a declaration on every page. The declaration is long and there will be at least 14 pages in each LPA document, so rather than risk spoiling the copies and causing frustration for the person with dementia, you may decide it's simpler to get the certified copies made at a solicitor's office, for a small fee for each one.

Enduring Power of Attorney

If the person you care for did some forward planning, they may already have an Enduring Power of Attorney (EPA) in place that names an attorney. If it was made and signed before October 2007, when EPAs were replaced by LPAs, it is still in force and you will still be able to use it – you do not have to do a new Lasting Power of Attorney. If the person who made the EPA is no longer able to manage their finances you must first register it with the Office of the Public Guardian.

EPAs were only designed to allow attorneys to help with financial matters, so you may still need to help the person with dementia complete an LPA for health and welfare if they wish to do this.

Using an LPA for property and finance

Banks and building societies differ in their procedures. Some will just ask to see the LPA (or EPA), or a certified copy, and make a note on their records and allow you to carry on using the person you care for's cheque book. (You will also be asked for proof of your identity.) Some will close the accounts in the person you care for's name and open new ones, entitled, for example, 'J Smith, LPA for Mrs M Smith'. If this is the case, new cheque or pass books will be issued for the account, along with new debit cards. You will also be offered online banking if you would like it.

Be prepared for things not to run smoothly. Banks and building societies are only just getting used to the increasing use of LPAs and not all bank staff are properly trained. This is something that the Office of the Public Guardian and the Financial Conduct Authority are working hard to address at the time of writing.

When we registered the LPA for my mother-in-law, the bank withdrew her debit card and would not issue one on the new account. When I enquired why, I was told that it was because, due to her mental incapacity, she might 'draw out all her money'. When I pointed out that it was her money and she was entitled to do so, they didn't really have an answer. They promised to write to me with an explanation but never did so.

You now have the power to set up and cancel direct debits and standing orders on behalf of the person you care for, to write cheques and to withdraw cash and spend it for the person's benefit. You also have the power to make cash gifts if this is something he/she would normally do. You must manage the money in a responsible manner and follow any instructions set out in the LPA.

Keep careful records of how you manage the person with dementia's money. The Court of Protection can ask to see your records at any time, although they seldom do so. Keep the person with dementia's money and financial affairs separate from your own – unless, of course, you are married and have a joint account.

Using an LPA for health and welfare

Once the person you care for is no longer able to make decisions about their health and welfare, you will need to contact their GP and other healthcare staff, their social care worker, care home staff, agency carers, friends and family – if they don't already know – and tell them that you are now the first point of contact. You may be asked to show the original LPA or a certified copy, and proof of your identity. When making decisions for the person with dementia, follow any notes in the LPA, and talk to friends and family about what the person would like. Aim to make decisions that are in the best interest of the person with dementia, not easy options that suit other people.

Note that if the person you care for has already made an Advance Directive (see below) and then later gives an LPA for health and welfare, then their previous Advance Directive is no longer valid – unless the LPA makes specific reference to using it.

When no LPA or EPA has been made

If the person you care for becomes mentally incapacitated and no LPA or EPA is in place you have to notify the Court of Protection. The Court of Protection will then appoint someone – called a deputy – to manage the affairs of the person with dementia. Typically this is a family member or close friend, but the court may appoint someone else – for example, a solicitor or the local authority. The court will tell the deputy which decisions they can or cannot make for the person with dementia. More guidance is available on the government website gov.uk or you can phone for an information pack (see reference section for details (page 211): the phone number is 0300 456 4600).

MAKING A WILL

Many people put off writing a Will because it seems morbid or because death seems so far away, or perhaps because they believe it might upset their close family. Many are also under the impression that if they do not write a Will 'my spouse/children/ family will get everything anyway'. However, this is not the case. If someone dies without leaving a Will (they die 'intestate') then the law has strict criteria about where the money goes and it may not be where the person you are caring for would choose.

If someone has dementia this does not mean that they can't make a Will, although they must be able to understand what they are doing.

Making a Will is not morbid and it is not a waste of time. On the contrary, making a Will is thoughtful and it is a kindness to those left behind. It shows that the person making the Will cared for them and for what will happen to them after his/her death. It takes pressure off loved ones at a time of grief and stress, and it means that the complicated paperwork after a death is simplified.

A Will does not have to be drawn up by a solicitor. It can be written by hand or printed. It can be written on a plain sheet of paper or on a 'Will form' bought from a stationers or a website. People tend to use a solicitor because they are afraid that they will not word things correctly or not be able to make their wishes clear. These are valid worries and if the person who is making the Will has complicated financial affairs, then it is better to use an expert to draft the document.

A Will must be signed and dated and the signature must be witnessed by two people who will not benefit from any bequests in it. It should name an 'executor' – the person who will make sure that the instructions in the Will are carried out. The executor can be a beneficiary of the Will. It is usual to ask someone if they are prepared to be an executor before appointing them; this can be a responsible and time-consuming job and not everyone will wish to take it on.

Many people think that it is safest to appoint a bank or a solicitor as the executor of a Will. This is not necessarily the wisest choice. Banks and solicitors will charge a fee to act as executor and this will reduce the dead person's 'estate' – sometimes considerably. It may also delay the proving of the Will and the dispersal of any money.

It is quite common, and perfectly legal, for husbands and wives to appoint each other as executor, but if one of you subsequently develops dementia, you will need to reconsider this. The person who is going to inherit the bulk of the estate can also be a good choice.

Some people lodge their Will with a bank or a solicitor for safe-keeping. Some people just store it with other important documents in the home. Make sure that you know where the person you care for keeps his/her Will. And make a Will yourself. You will want to make sure that if you die first, the person you care for will be looked after.

If someone develops dementia after they have been appointed as an executor, then it is important that you inform the person who has made the Will so that they can appoint another executor. It would be very unfair to place the burden of being executor of a Will on someone who has dementia and it is unlikely that they would be able to carry out all, or possibly any, of the duties correctly.

ADVANCE STATEMENTS AND ADVANCE DECISIONS

Sometimes people think ahead and wish to make their views about their care known in case of a diagnosis of dementia. An Advance Statement is a way of doing this: it covers preferences for medical and other treatments and personal lifestyle preferences and it can be referred to when the person with dementia is no longer able to discuss what they would like to happen.

Although doctors and other medical professionals may take into account the views stated in an Advance Statement, they are not legally bound to if they believe that it is not in the person's best interests from a medical point of view.

An Advance Decision is something separate. It sets out under which conditions a person wishes to refuse life-sustaining treatment. It IS legally binding in England and Wales and doctors must follow its instructions.

People can make an Advance Statement and an Advance Decision if they want to.

Advance Statements

As well as medical treatment preferences, an Advance Statement can include views and preferences on domestic arrangements, finances, information disclosure, how pets should be looked after, and diet options, for example. It can name someone with whom medical treatment might be discussed if the person making the statement is not able to do this. It might specify the desire to die at home.

Vegetarians might wish to state that they want to be offered vegetarian food after they've lost the capacity to remind carers that they don't eat meat. People who are unable to speak might like to specify with whom they would prefer their welfare to be discussed.

An Advance Statement can be seen as a 'negative' document, but making such a statement can have very positive effects. It can act as a safeguard and offer protection from neglect, as individuals can record their wishes for life to be sustained by any reasonable means and for pain relief to be given whenever required.

An Advance Statement is sometimes called a 'personal values history' or a 'living will' and it can help health professionals and family and close friends to decide what sort of treatment a person might want if for some reason they are unable to communicate their wishes. However, an Advance Statement does not bind healthcare professionals to a particular course of action and they may not carry out treatment if it conflicts with their professional judgement.

Advance Decisions

An Advance Decision specifically allows the person making it to state under what conditions he/she chooses to refuse life-sustaining treatment. So, for example, they may state that they do not wish to be fed or hydrated artificially if there is no reasonable hope of recovery. It is possible to refuse resuscitation in certain circumstances. Healthcare professionals are legally bound to follow an Advance Decision refusing treatment (but see the note above about any subsequent LPA for health and welfare overriding this unless specifically declared not to).

An Advance Decision cannot be used to ask for anything that is illegal, such as euthanasia; to refuse food or drink by mouth; or to refuse measures that are meant solely to maintain comfort, such as providing pain relief or warmth or personal care.

The Advance Decision does not allow the person making it to state what treatment they would like, only what treatment they refuse – hence many people make an Advance Decision and an Advance Statement (see above). It must also be worded more specifically than an Advance Statement and it must meet certain requirements set out in the Mental Capacity Act. Life-sustaining treatment is defined in the Act as treatment which, in the view of the person providing the healthcare, is necessary to sustain the patient's life.

There are legal requirements for a valid Advance Decision to refuse life-sustaining treatment:

- The person making the Advance Decision must have the mental capacity to do so.
- The Advance Decision must be in writing. If the person making it is unable to write, they can ask someone else to do so.
- The Advance Decision must be signed. Again, if the person making it is unable to write in order to sign it, they can ask someone else to do so.
- The signature must be witnessed and the witness must sign the document in the presence of the person making it.
- The Advance Decision must include a written statement that says it applies to the specific treatment being refused <u>even if the person's life is at risk.</u>

An Advance Decision to refuse treatment must indicate exactly what type of treatment is being refused and should give as much detail as possible about the circumstances under which refusal would apply. It is not necessary to use medical terms or language, as long as it is clear.

What is the point?

As a carer, you may wonder whether there is any need or any point in the person with dementia making either an Advance Statement or an Advance Decision. They are not compulsory and doctors and other medical professionals will make the decisions that they feel to be in the person you care for's best interests according to circumstances at the time. They should still take into account any evidence they may have of the person's wishes and consult with family, friends and carers.

No one should feel under pressure to make either an Advance Statement or an Advance Decision. If you are caring for someone with dementia, neither of you should feel that this has to be done. It is entirely the person's decision whether to do so or not.

It is a waste of time if the person with dementia makes an Advance Statement or an Advance Decision if no one knows about it or where it is kept, so make sure relevant people have the details. It is also wise to make several copies. Give one to the person with dementia's GP and ask for it to be attached to their medical notes. Keep a spare copy to be attached to hospital notes if necessary. Any new medical staff that come into contact with the person you are caring for are unlikely to be aware of any Advance Decision or Statement, so be prepared to draw their attention to this. And don't assume that hospital staff will always read the person's medical notes before they treat them.

(See also chapter 3 for information on care plans and 'hospital passports'.)

END-OF-LIFE WISHES

We all have our own ideas and wishes (however vaguely they are acknowledged) about how we would like the last days of our life to be managed. Some people will have written these wishes down. When people with dementia move to a residential care home, part of the admissions procedure should include noting their wishes for end-of-life care and keeping these with their care plan.

As a carer, you can make sure that the person you look after has recorded their end-of-life wishes and keeps them in a safe place known to you. Some carers won't have discussed this aspect with the person they care for, and if you have left it too late in the illness to do so, you as the carer and the person closest to them are the most likely person to understand what their wishes may be. At this stage, be sure that anything recorded is as near as possible to what you think is truly the wish of the person you are caring for – rather than reflecting what you yourself want for them. For example, you may feel that a person with dementia has a very low quality of life and that it is not worth preserving at any cost – it is easy to project our own strongly felt wishes on someone who is unable to express their own opinion.

Care homes must make an end-of-life plan that takes account of the individual resident's wishes; they should record whether the resident wants to be resuscitated and under what circumstances. 'Do not recuscitate', or 'Allow natural death', should not appear on medical notes unless this has been previously requested by the resident and/or agreed with their family.

Many people with dementia have strong feelings about whether they might die in hospital. Many care homes are willing to allow someone to spend their last days in the place that is now their home, rather than in the strange and confusing atmosphere of a hospital, provided the home's medical staff agree.

It may seem difficult to face up to many of these practical matters when you are already having to come to terms with the reality of a diagnosis of dementia. However, sorting things out before they become urgent can give you and the person with dementia some peace of mind.

Chapter 12

Caring for yourself

Caring for yourself is essential both for you and for the person who depends on you. If you are ill, exhausted or depressed, you cannot look after them as you would like. Do not feel guilty about asking for help and do not let things get so bad there is a crisis you could have seen coming. A contented carer is a good carer and it is worth remembering the person with dementia remembers the emotions you show much more than the words you use.

Being a carer is stressful and tiring. It can also be very fulfilling and many of us are glad to be 'giving something back', especially if it is to a parent who once cared for us. However, there is no denying that caring for someone with dementia can sometimes feel as though we are labouring under an intolerable burden. It is very seldom, even in the best regulated and closest of families, that the burden of caring is shared equally amongst the family members. There may be many reasons for this. Some members of the family may live too far away to give 'hands on' care. Some may have a closer relationship with the person being cared for. Some people work longer hours or in more stressful jobs. Sometimes, sadly, family members just do not want to be involved in the care of their relatives. Frequently, the burden of care falls on the family member or friend (if family are not involved) who lives nearest, or who is seen as having the most time to give. With dementia, male partners and sons may be involved as carers just as often as female partners and daughters.

In general, the role of 'carer' is not planned for or logically decided upon. Dementia almost always begins slowly and imperceptibly and people do not normally awake to find that they have become a 'carer' overnight. A spouse or partner or a child will just gradually find themselves managing more areas of the life of someone who is cognitively impaired: a husband perhaps begins to help organise the cooking, a wife may start to manage the money when she previously left it to her husband, a son or daughter may find that they have to organise car servicing or shopping.

On the other hand, people may fall ill suddenly, accidents may happen, there may be an unexpected death, or some other event may overtake us, and the role of carer may suddenly be ours without planning or forethought. Very often there is a dramatic change after the death of one member of an elderly couple. There is a sudden realisation that the remaining partner will not be able to cope alone without substantial input from other members of the family, or friends – 'the carers'. In such an emergency, contingency plans have to be made and actions taken without time to consider the consequences.

If at all possible, make time after the initial 'emergency' to take a step back, draw breath and make a care plan. It is very worthwhile at this stage to get everyone together and agree a plan. Lack of this sort of co-operation may turn out to be the biggest underlying problem later on. Resentment and hostility quickly build up in the absence of communication. Guilt plays a part. A daughter living at some distance away may really resent the 'hands on' care given by a daughter-in-law, even though she knows that she is unable to give it herself. A son may not feel at all able to give this kind of care and react by belittling the care given by his sisters. This is the time to organise a 'team' (see chapter 2 page 21).

Don't try to go it alone

If you are the only available family member, don't try to take
on everything alone. There may well be neighbours or friends
of the person you are caring for who will help in the same way
that family do. If not, you will need professional help. There is
no need to feel guilty about this. Indeed, some people with dementia prefer the notion that any help they are receiving is 'paid'
help and not done as a favour. Remember that you do not have
to go through social services to get professional help, although
you may wish to do so.

Caring for a member of the family is an unpaid occupation
but you, or the person you care for, may be able to claim certain
grants and allowances. If you are entitled to them, you should
certainly claim them. Do not allow the person you care for, or
yourself, to be put off by thoughts of 'living off the state' or
claiming 'charity'. Most of us have paid into the state through
National Insurance contributions and taxes, and all of us are
entitled to claim help from the state when we need it.

There is an additional factor. Being in receipt of certain benefits
often qualifies you for other financial help or gives you priority
when seeking other 'non-cash' benefits. Some benefits are means
tested and the entitlement may in itself mean very little. You
may think that the receipt of say 40 pence per week is not worth
the effort of claiming, but the extra benefits associated with it
may make it very worthwhile. An example of this is Attendance
Allowance, which may entitle someone to a reduction in Council
tax payments (see Chapter 11 on Practical matters – page 178).

Get a carer's assessment for yourself

You may also not realise that if you are a carer, you can ask the
local authority – through the social care team – for an assessment
of your own needs (see also Chapter 3, page 43). If you live in

England or Wales you are entitled to an assessment whether or not the person you are caring for is having an assessment themselves. In Scotland you can only receive an assessment if the person you are caring for is being assessed. Except in Scotland, where there is no standard list of what should be assessed, the assessment is supposed to take into account your work or desire to work and your need for training, education and leisure activities.

The kind of help and support you can get as a carer includes: respite care to give you a break if you are caring constantly for someone else; emotional support from other carers, usually through a local support group; help with caring; and help with household tasks and activities for the person you care for. You should also be told about any benefits you are entitled to claim. Your assessment may be made by a social worker from the local authority social services department, or it may be carried out by a worker from a private agency employed on behalf of social services. It may be made over the telephone. Before you have an assessment you might want to think about the following points:

- If you need to get up in the night to care for someone, are you getting enough sleep?
- Are you able to get out and do things by yourself or does the person you care for need to have someone with them constantly?
- Do you feel that your health is being affected by caring? For example, do you have to do any heavy lifting (physical health) or is the situation making you depressed (mental health)?
- Are you able to cope with other family commitments? For example, do you also have to run a home and care for your spouse and children?
- Are you finding it difficult to juggle working for a living and caring? You may be having to work to earn a living and trying to fit caring in around your working day.

Talk to the person doing your assessment about these and any other issues that you think may affect your ability to continue caring. Remember that by caring for your relative or friend you are helping to maintain the current state policy of ensuring 'care in the community' and are saving the state money.

If you feel that you need an urgent assessment (if you suddenly have to go into hospital, for example) then get in touch with the social services duty officer because they are able to organise an emergency assessment.

Look for sources of help far and wide

Carers are a huge 'silent force' within the community and many struggle on feeling that to ask for help is a confession of weakness and inability to cope. In a perfect world we would receive all the help needed to care for someone through official channels and all the facilities would be there to assist us. In actual fact, the level of help available varies widely from area to area. Local authorities have limited resources and have to give the help they can to those most in need, based on their own assessment of where the need is greatest. So it is fairly certain that you yourself will have to find ways and means to relieve some of the burden of caring.

First, do not avoid asking your friends and neighbours for help if you need it (see Chapter 2 on 'building your team'). They may well be able and willing to fill 'gaps' in the help supplied officially. Many people are pleased and even flattered to be asked to help, but the most important advice here is to be specific about what you ask– see chapter 2 for more on this.

A neighbour will often promise to 'keep an eye on things', but it would be much more useful if you asked them to do something specific – say, *'Can you call round each morning just to check all is well?'* or *'Could you be a second key holder for the call alarm?'* Of course, people may sometimes be unable to help but unless and until you ask you will never know.

199

*I was having trouble keeping up with the laundry as I did not
have a tumble dryer and the weather was so bad. One day I was
grumbling about this to my support worker and she suggested
I ask a neighbour whether they could help. I was amazed to find
that two of my neighbours were most happy to dry laundry loads
for me. One of them said she had been 'racking her brain' trying
to think of how to help me.*

Check for available help at local clubs and organisations that
the person you care for belongs to. If he or she belongs to a
church you will almost certainly be able to get lifts to church
services and any church-related clubs. You may also get offers
of respite in the form of visitors or help with shopping and
other errands. If the person you care for belongs to a local
branch of an organisation, such as the British Legion or the
Rotary Club, ask if members can offer any help. Ex-service men
and women's organisations can be particularly helpful; many
elderly people are ex-services or did National Service after the
Second World War.

Another source of help can be local branches of organisations
set up to benefit ex-members of professions or trades. Use the
local library or the internet as a starting point. Some organisations have holiday care hotels that offer respite for people with
dementia and their carers.

Local and national charities can also be sources of help. You
may think that your needs, or those of the person you care for,
are too insignificant to be of interest to these charities, but you
may be surprised to learn that some charities, far from having
their resources stretched too thinly, are desperate to find those
who need their help.

My friend was temporary Chief Executive of a charity that helped those who could not afford to pay their water charges. He surprised me by telling me one day that the charity had great trouble finding people to help, not because the help was not needed but because their advertising was poor and people who needed their help simply didn't know it was available for the asking.

Dealing with guilt

Although it can be very difficult, try not to allow yourself to feel constantly guilty. Those we care for do not always show their appreciation, and indeed, in some cases, they may be unable to do so. Parents have grown used to nagging their children, old friends have grown used to taking help given for granted. Other members of the family may find it easier to find fault with the care you are giving rather than offer support. Reassure yourself that you are doing the best you can. Do not feel guilty if you sometimes feel annoyed with or speak crossly to someone you care for. If you feel that your feelings may get the better of you and lead to any form of action stronger than cross words, make every attempt to stand back from the situation and seek help. Support organisations and social care teams will understand your feelings and not condemn you for them.

Look after your own health

It is very important that you look after your own physical and mental health. Take care of yourself physically by eating properly and getting some exercise.. You should never neglect your own health issues – you owe this to yourself and to the person you care for. As you will be aware, if you become ill the person you are caring for will suffer too, as you won't be able to look after them properly.

If you visit your doctor for a health problem that needs a referral to an outpatient clinic or an operation, make sure that the doctor knows you are a carer. When referring patients, doctors take into account not only the severity of the health problem referred but also any circumstances in the patient's life that might mean they should be seen more quickly than normal. This is standard practice, but your doctor cannot take the fact that you are a carer into account if he/she doesn't know about it.

These days most doctors do not know their patients personally and, although they should ask you about problems at home that might be affecting your health, many do not have time to do so. So tell the doctor that you are a carer and that you will need to make special arrangements for the person you look after in order to get treatment for your own health. You can now obtain a form that enables you to record the fact that you are a carer with the doctor. The form is available from the receptionist at your GP surgery, in public libraries and Citizen's Advice Bureaux and through many carers' agencies. Complete the form and hand it to your doctor so that it can be kept with your medical notes.

You need a break from time to time

If you are a full-time carer you should do your very best to build some 'respite' time into your daily life. You should not consider respite as a selfish option, nor should you feel guilty about it. You are the main carer, you are bearing most of the burden (however willing you may be to bear it) and you are the most important person in the life of the person you are looking after. Make no mistake here – people with dementia often behave most badly with the person who is closest to them, but they do so precisely because they are secure in your loving care. **You are the person**

who is most important to them so it is essential that you take a lot of care of yourself.

You cannot give of your best in any situation if you are tired, harassed and bad tempered, ill or in need of rest. Periods of rest are essential. Rest, in this context, means a rest from the constant caring – it does not necessarily mean rest from activity.

Most of us who are constantly caring feel that we need some space in our lives every day. Some people will be able to fit this into the course of the daily routine. Others (especially those couples who have always done 'everything together') will find this more difficult. If you are caring for a person with dementia who does not live with you (such as a parent, for example) you will have periods in the day when you are not with them physically – although the weight of caring for them may seem never to lift from your shoulders.

Practical ways to take a break

Try to plan for a short time to yourself each day. You may be able to take advantage of the fact that the person with dementia goes to bed earlier or wakes later than you do. In the earlier stages of the illness, the person with dementia may still take short outings alone – walking the dog or going to the shop – and this may be your time to yourself. However, you may have to plan this time specifically by asking someone else to take over. Do not think that a short time each day is not worth having. You will find that it is important.

You might pay for a carer to come in and sit with the person you look after for a couple of hours once or twice a week, or you might be able to find a friend, neighbour or other family member who will do this. You may find a local charity or other organisation which will provide this kind of service. You could make use of a day-centre service on one or more days each week so that you can plan your own activities on those days.

If you are regularly woken at night in order to care for your relative or friend, then for your own health you should try to organise at least one night of unbroken sleep each week. There are agencies which provide a 'night sitting' service, or you could ask another member of the family to give you relief from night duty on a regular basis.

Arrange a proper holiday for yourself

When you are caring for someone with dementia full time you may want to go away on holiday without the person you care for occasionally, as a form of respite. Another member of the family, or a friend or neighbour, may be prepared to take over your visiting and caring duties for the length of the holiday. The fact is that families can sometimes be quite selfish over this and so you may have to be prepared to be insistent.

Another option is to try to arrange respite care for your relative or friend in a local care or nursing home. Although theoretically many homes offer this facility, some will only do so if they happen to have a free bed – not all homes keep permanent 'respite' beds. Therefore, your chosen home may not have room at the time you need it.

The person you care for may also be quite stubborn about going away for respite care. They may be worried that it is 'the thin end of the wedge', leading up to a permanent placement in a care home, which they may dread. They may just not want to leave their familiar surroundings. Familiarity is an important element of independence for people with dementia. As explained in chapter 1 – About dementia – those who have dementia may lose their ability to empathise and it will be hard to make them understand that you need a break from caring. They may respond by saying that they can manage perfectly well alone. It may be possible to try to enlist the help of other family members to persuade the person you care for that you need the break.

However, it may be necessary simply to go ahead and make the arrangements for respite care, remembering that you are acting in the best interests of the person you care for. Don't forget that the local authority social services department has a 'duty of care' for carers; if you are struggling to make informal arrangements or can't find a local care/nursing home to help, contact the duty officer in the social services department.

When making arrangements for respite you should limit explanations to a clear and simple statement of what is going to happen, coupled with reassurances that things will return to normal in time; that is, you will return home if you are going out or that the person you care for will come back home after the period of respite care is over. You should not show that you are worried or upset, even if you have real concerns. Remember that the person with dementia remembers the emotion you show much more than the words you use.

Join a support group

There are several organisations aimed at supporting carers and your support worker, local library, GP surgery or district nursing team can put you in touch with these. You can also find information about local groups via the internet. Some of these offer information, some offer practical support and some offer 'moral support' in the form of local support groups where carers can meet to talk about their problems or concerns with people who are in a similar situation to themselves.

Information about national carers' organisations can be obtained via the internet or again from your local library.

Many support organisations have online chat rooms and forums accessed via their website and you may find this kind of 'virtual' support most helpful as it can be accessed outside working hours, when you may actually have more time available.

Keep in touch with your friends

Caring for someone with dementia can be a full-time job and you may not realise that you are gradually losing your own social life and sense of self. You may sometimes feel very tired and come to believe that rest is more important than leisure activities or seeing your own friends. However, it is important that you continue to enjoy at least some of the activities you used to do before.

Where couples have lived together for many years it is often the case that they have fallen into the way of doing most things together socially. Some couples are unable to conceive the idea of a separate social life. While your partner is able to continue to enjoy the things you have always done together, the best thing both for you and for the person with dementia is to continue to do so. You may have to make some modifications if the person with dementia is unable to take part in particular activities, but often you can continue to enjoy an active joint social life.

If this is no longer possible, then it is reasonable and good, both for your health and for that of the person with dementia, that you have a separate social life. You may wish to go out to meet friends, to go to a carers' support group, to participate in a hobby or attend a club and there is no reason why you should feel guilty or unhappy about doing this, provided you have made sure that the person you are caring for is well looked after in your absence.

It can even be a good idea to take up a new interest that will give you a fresh opportunity to see yourself as more than just a carer. Although this may be difficult to imagine soon after the person you care for's diagnosis, it can be worth keeping in the back of your mind – if the person with dementia goes into full-time care later, you may need something to occupy your time and 'fill the gap' as your caring duties become less time-consuming.

It is essential for your own well-being to continue to have social relationships, to enjoy your hobbies and visit your friends as before. All the suggestions previously given about using your 'team', including friends, neighbours and professional carers, apply here. You should certainly not feel that you are being self-indulgent by continuing to enjoy a social life or personal hobbies and pastimes even if, as sometimes happens, the person with dementia makes difficulties or expresses their anxiety when you leave them with others.

Caring for parents with dementia

Children of people with dementia may often feel pulled all ways by the demands of their own partners and children or find it really difficult to carry on with their working life due to the added stress and guilt of caring for a parent. It can be a great privilege to care for an ageing parent and many of us are glad to do so, but it is equally important to maintain our own life.

Dementia can put a great strain on the parent-child relationship, even when it has been harmonious in the past. However, not everyone has enjoyed a good relationship with their parents and some people can find themselves the unwilling carer of a parent with whom they do not get on, forced through circumstance into a relationship from which they thought they had escaped. This can cause a tremendous amount of stress, guilt and even feelings amounting almost to hatred – in both the carer and the person being cared for.

If you are in this unfortunate position, it is even more important that you do not try to do everything yourself. You can remind yourself that an unwilling carer is not the best carer and make full use of professional agencies and anyone else in your caring 'team'. Do not think that your support workers and social care workers will not understand. They are professional people who will have had a wide experience of problems experienced by carers and they will be best placed to help you if you are honest with them about what you feel you are able to do and what you do not feel able to do. Employers and partners/spouses can be very supportive and helpful in these circumstances, but equally they can add to the burden when they are not understanding and supportive.

CONCLUSION

Most of this book is about how to care for someone with dementia but in this chapter I have endeavoured to explain how important it is to care for yourself. This can be very difficult to do when caring gradually takes up more and more of your time and when you may begin to feel very isolated. Remember that help is out there in the form of dementia advisers and support workers, social care workers, carers' support groups and, hopefully, the friends and family who form part of your caring team. You are a very important person in the life of the person you care for and you should always remind yourself that you are worth caring for too.

Appendix

Further useful information

Alzheimer societies in the English-speaking world

Alzheimer's Society
Tel: +44 (0)20 7423 3500
Website: www.alzheimers.org.uk

Alzheimer's Research UK
Tel: +44 (0) 300 111 5555
Website: www.alzheimersresearchuk.org/

Alzheimer Society of Ireland
Tel: +353 (01) 207 3800
Website: www.alzheimer.ie

Alzheimer's Scotland
Tel: +44 (0)808 808 3000 (helpline)
Website: www.alzscot.org

Alzheimer's Australia
Tel: +61 1800 100 500 (helpline)
Website: www.fightdementia.org.au

Alzheimer Society Canada
Tel: +1 416-488-8772
Website: www.alzheimer.ca

Alzheimer's Association (USA)
Tel: +1 800-272-3900
Website: www.alz.org

Dementia societies

Dementia Research Centre
Tel: +44 (0)20 3448 4773
Website: www.ucl.ac.uk/drc

Dementia UK
Tel: +44 (0) 20 7697 4160
Website: www.dementiauk.org/

Dementia Services Information and Development Centre, Ireland
Tel: +353 1 416 2035
Website: www.dementia.ie

Diabetes societies

Diabetes UK
Tel: +44 (0) 345 123 2399
Website: www.diabetes.org.uk

Diabetes Australia
Tel: + 61 (02) 6232 3800
Website: www.diabetesaustralia.com.au

Diabetes Ireland
Tel: 1850 909 909 (helpline)
http://www.diabetes.ie/

Canadian Diabetes Association
Tel: +1 416-363-3373
Website: www.diabetes.ca

American Diabetes Association
Tel: +1-800-342-2383 (helpline)
Website: www.diabetes.org

Public services

Information about UK government services, tax, benefits and pensions and other government-regulated financial matters such as power of attorney can now all be found on one central website: www.gov.uk

Department of Work and Pensions
www.gov.uk/government/organisations/department-for-work-pensions

Office of the Public Guardian
For information about Power of Attorney
Tel: 0300 456 0300
www.justice.gov.uk/about/opg

Power of Attorney, Ireland
Relevant legislation in Ireland is the Power of Attorney Act 1996 and the Enduring Powers of Attorney Regulations (Statutory Instrument No 196/1996)
One useful source of information is:
The Faculty of Notaries Public in Ireland
Tel: +353 (0)1 497 3611
Website: www.notarypublic.ie

Sources of support

Action on Hearing Loss
Online shop with aids for everyday living for the deaf
Tel: 0808 808 0123
Textphone: 0808 808 9000
www.actiononhearingloss.org.uk

Age UK
Tel: +44 (0)800 169 6565 (advice line)
www.ageuk.org.uk

Age Action Ireland
Promotes positive ageing and better policies and services for older people.
Tel: 01 4756989
www.ageaction.ie

Carers Trust
Tel: +44 (0)844 800 4361
Website: www.carers.org

Carers UK
Tel: +44 (0)808 808 7777
Website: www.carersuk.org

The Carers Association
For family carers in Ireland
Tel: 1800 240724 (helpline)
www.carersireland.com

Disability Rights UK (RADAR)
Tel: +44 (0)20 7250 3222
Website: www.radar-shop.org.uk

Disabled Living Foundation
Provides information and advice on equipment. There is an Equipment Demonstration Centre with large displays of equipment which visitors can try out and where advice can be obtained.
Helpline: 0300 999 0004 (charged at local call rate)
Equipment Demonstration Centre: (020) 7289 6111 ext 247
Website: www.dlf.org.uk

RNIB – Royal National Institute for the Blind
Tel: 0303 123 9999
Website: www.rnib.org.uk/

Royal Voluntary Service (RVS)
Meals-on-wheels and social transport schemes; a good-neighbour scheme for minor household repairs
Tel: 0845 600 5885
Website: www.royalvoluntaryservice.org.uk

Think Ahead, Ireland
For guidance on recording preferences in the event of emergency, serious illness or death
Tel: +353 (0)1 679 3188
Website: www.thinkahead.ie

Sources of useful products

Assist UK Disabled Living Centres
A network of centres around the UK which provides information and advice on products and where you can see and try out products.
Tel: 0161 832 9757
Website: http://assist-uk.org

British Red Cross
Ability Catalogue – products for independence
Tel: 0844 89 300 90
Website: www.redcross.org.uk

Incontinence Products
Tel: 0800 051 7729
Website: www.dryforlife.co.uk

Lloyds Pharmacy
Local pharmacy branches stock catalogues of aids and equipment
and can order items for you and have them delivered to your nearest pharmacy. The website has a 'nearest pharmacy' search facility.
Website: www.lloydspharmacy.co.uk

Independent Living
Provides impartial information for family carers, care professionals and individuals with a disability, about products and services
to help with mobility and independence.
Website: www.independentliving.co.uk

Stannah
UK's biggest provider of stairlifts
Tel: 0808 256 4910
Website: www.stannah.com

Uniscan Walkers
Provider of a variety of 'walkers'
Tel: 01268 419 288
Website: www.uniscan-walkers.co.uk

Wiltshire Farm Foods
Deliver frozen ready-meals to your home
Tel: 0800 773 773
www.wiltshirefarmfoods.com

Sources of financial advice

Citizens Advice Bureaux, UK
The Citizens Advice service helps people resolve their legal, financial and other problems by providing free, independent and confidential advice.
Local telephone numbers can be found on their website or via direc-
tory inquiries.
Website: www.citizensadvice.org.uk

Citizens Information Board, Ireland
Centres throughout the country; contact details at:
Website: www.citizensinformation.ie

Co-Operative Mobility
This site enables you to assess yourself for Disability Living Allowance or Attendance Allowance before you apply. You can find out whether you qualify and at what rate you are likely to be paid.
Tel: 0845 459 6006
Website: www.co-operativeindependentliving.co.uk/

Foundations
Information on local home improvement agencies to help older people stay in their own homes.
Tel: 0845 864 5210
Website: www.foundations.uk.com

Independent Age
Aims to provide lifelong support for the elderly on very low incomes.
Tel: 0800 319 6789
Website: www.independentage.org

Care Home fees planning
Time Independent Ltd
Tel: 0118 327 9895
http://www.carehomefeesplanning.co.uk/

Transport and mobility

Department for Transport, UK
General information about transport facilities for the elderly
Website: www.gov.uk/government/organisations/department-for-transport

Blue Badge scheme
To obtain a 'disabled' parking badge in the UK
Telephone numbers differ – badge issued by local councils.
Website: www.gov.uk/browse/disabilities

Disabled Parking Permit Scheme, Ireland
To get a parking card you must apply through the Disabled Drivers Association of Ireland:
Website: www.ddai.ie
or the Irish Wheelchair Association
Website: www.iwa.ie

Application forms must be signed by your doctor and counter-signed by a Garda.
The parking card must be reviewed every two years.

Health and health professionals

British Association of Occupational Therapists
Tel: 020 7357 6480
Website: www.cot.co.uk

Association of Occupational Therapists of Ireland
Tel: +353 (01) 874 8136
Website: www.aoti.ie

The Outside Clinic
Offers eye tests and an eye care service in your own home
Tel: 0800 85 4477
Website: www.outsideclinic.com

Visioncall UK and Ireland
Home-visiting opticians in Ireland and UK and can provide a free home eye test at your convenience.
Tel: 0845 050 1831
Website: www.vision-call.co.uk

Telecare
Tel: 0300 123 1002 (free leaflet)
Website: www.nhs.uk/Planners/Yourhealth/Pages/Telecare.aspx

IrishHealth.com
Official online source of health information in Ireland.

Index

Index

bath or shower, 32, 43, 71, 84, 92, 104–105, 109
behaviour (cared-for), xi, 55–68
    clinging and demanding, 67–68
    in residential homes, 70–73
    unacceptable, 65–66, 92, 107–109
    see also inhibition
behaviour (carer), xii, 97–110
benefits and allowances, 178–181
blood sugar, low, 6
Blue Badge scheme, 214
books, 136–137
boredom, 59, 66, 135–141
brain, 14–16
    communication and the, 77
    executive function, 3, 84, 111, 161
    glucose and the, 156
    socialising and the, 160
    stroke and the, 165–166
breakfast, 81, 90, 115
breaks *see* respite and breaks
British Association of Occupational Therapists, 215
British Red Cross, 212
bullying, 107–109
burden of care, 141, 195–196
Butterfly Scheme, 49

Canada
    Alzheimer's Society, 209
    Diabetes Association, 210
care
    burden of, 141, 195–196
    duty of, 53, 205
    professional *see* professionals
care homes (residential/nursing homes), 29, 68–74
    end-of-life care in, 193, 194
    fees, 181–182, 214
    respite care in, 29, 204
    specialist (in dementia), 69–70, 71
    staff *see* staff
carers
    allowance, 180–181
    caring for themselves, 195–208
    needs *see* needs
Carers Association, 212
Carers Trust, 211
Carers UK, 211

charities, 200–201, 203
    see also voluntary support organisations
chest infections, 164, 169–170
child (of parent with dementia)
    relationship with parent, 207
    reluctance to ask for support from, 23
cholinesterase inhibitors, 17
Citizens Advice Board (Ireland), 213
Citizens Advice Bureaux, 42, 179, 181, 202, 213
clinging behaviour, 67–68
clothing and dressing, 6, 11, 79, 113–115
clue-giving *see* prompts and clue-giving
coconut oil, 157
cognitive impairment/problems, 97
    concern and worries about possible existence of, 36–37
    hospital stay-related, 46–47, 53
    mild, 2, 9–10
colds, 164, 169–170
communication, 75–95
    avoiding contradiction, 102–103
    hearing loss and, 173
    problems, xii, 75–95
    tips for success, 87
community mental health team, 38–39
community psychiatric nurses (CPNs), 39, 65, 172
confusion
    stroke and, 167
    urinary infection and, 168, 169
Constant Attendance Allowance, 180
consultant psychiatrist, 37, 38, 39
continence problems, 62–63, 169, 213
contradiction, avoiding, 102–103
convalescence, 52–53
conversation speed, 77–78
cooking, 12, 29, 138, 155–156, 157
Co-Operative Mobility, 214
Council Tax Disregard, 180
couples, dementia in one partner, 22–23, 206
Court of Protection, 182, 187
cries for help, 89–92
criticism, avoiding, 103–104
cursing, 92

Index

Index

Index

About the author

Mary Jordan has experience on both sides of dementia care – as a carer to friends and relatives, and professionally through her work for a national dementia charity; she daily supports people with a diagnosis of dementia, together with their carers. For many years she worked for the National Health Service and has also served in the Armed Forces. In addition to articles and papers published in medical, nursing and social care journals, she is also known for her books *The Fundholder's Handbook*, the award winning *End of Life – the essential guide to caring*, *The Essential Guide to Avoiding Dementia*, and *The Essential Carer's Guide*.

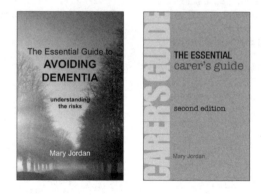

See:

www.maryjordan.co.uk for further information about all Mary's books

www.adaptdementia.com for more information about all the subject areas covered in the *Essential Carer's Guide to Dementia*, including counselling services and training.